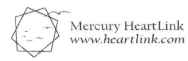

Mercury HeartLink
www.heartlink.com

AUTISM
A Dad's Journey

AUTISM

A Dad's Journey

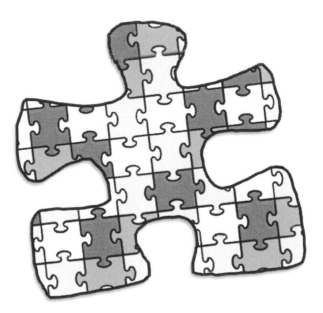

LUIS M. BAYARDO

Autism: A Dad's Journey
Copyright ©2014 Luis M. Bayardo

ISBN: 978-1-940769-16-5
Publisher: Mercury HeartLink
Printed in the United States of America

Autism: A Dad's Journey website:
www.autismadadsjourney.com

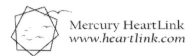

Mercury HeartLink
www.heartlink.com

Contents

Appendices

Acknowledgments

Over the course of the past 16 years so many professionals, therapists, and teachers have moved through our lives helping us on our incredible journey with our boys. We will be forever in your debt for your contributions to their phenomenal progress. A special thanks to Paula for encouraging me to share a father's view.

Donna (my mother-in-law) and Carol, thank you for helping me get the final draft ready for presentation. It would not have passed muster without your help. Donna you truly are an angel and the best mother-in-law I could have ever asked for. I love you.

Kim, thank you for suggesting I un-sterilize my thoughts and emotions. Without your suggestions I would never have shared my intimate thoughts and feelings that are so critical in this book.

Phil, thanks for your unique insights in making me feel this book was worth finishing and your thoughts on some final touches.

Brenna, thank you for all your help and support and your awesome ideas for the cover page.

Last but most importantly I must thank my wife Dana for making this book a reality. Although her name is not on the book cover, it would not have seen the light of day without her tireless dedication to its compilation and completion. I wrote the following chapters one paragraph, one thought, and one memory at a time over the course of a year. It took her dogged determination to turn these random thoughts into the cohesive picture of my Journey chronicled in the following pages. Dana is not only the hero of our marriage but also the inspiration for my existence. Without her I would not be whole. I love you Dana Corinne.

To my children, that make my life full:
Brenna, Kyler, Koleden, and Taylee Shea.

To all the parents who fight every day
to help their special children reach their full potential.

To my eternal companion, Dana Corinne,
thank you for walking beside me on my journey.

AUTISM

A Dad's Journey

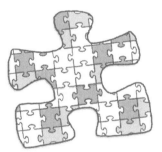

PREFACE

Although this is my story, this book is not about me but instead the journey many fathers must take. I am like most men. I am private, stoic, generally unemotional, and basically believe in keeping my private life to myself. I keep my thoughts and feelings buried deep within and hidden not only from those around me but often even from myself. I have chosen to share these intimate dark places not for my own edification but to give fathers like me a voice so that others can get a glimpse into the life we live. When reading these pages, remove me and place any father of a special needs child in my place. It is my hope that after reading this book you will understand him just a little better.

I'm not a famous person, author, academician, doctor, athlete, or any other person of great public consequence. I am simply a husband and a father of four wonderful children, two girls and two boys. The boys just happen to have autism. My oldest son is more severe on the spectrum than my youngest. This said, regardless of the severity of this affliction, those families in a similar situation should know that this diagnosis will affect the rest of their lives in ways they may have just begun to fathom

Getting your head around what the diagnosis of autism will mean to you and your loved ones can be a daunting and overwhelming emotional roller coaster. The what, where, when, and most importantly why, will fill most of your thoughts and concerns on a daily basis. In the digital age we now live in, your first step might be to log on to the internet and start reading. The internet is so pervasive with information that you might go into "information overload." This will most likely be your first foray into an epidemic that will turn your entire world upside down. It will also start you, and those around you, on a journey of discovery of yourself and of the things you will need to do to assist your loved one in living as fulfilling and meaningful life as possible.

The diagnosis of my oldest son came at precisely the same time as the first major crossroad of my professional career. I had recently completed my schooling with a degree in hospitality management. This, coupled with my past 8 years of experience in the industry made me feel I was ready to start moving up the corporate ladder. Job offers were rolling in from around the country and things were looking up financially for my growing family. My wife Dana and I had finally come to the end of that tunnel of schooling, and we felt we had made the down payment on our professional dues. We were ready for the transition into a "regular life." I had the opportunity to get my start in the hospitality industry while working at the 16th Century Castle Mona Hotel on the Isle of Man in the United Kingdom. With this beginning it was my hope to follow in my mentor's footsteps and become an International Hospitality Trouble Shooter, traveling around the world every few years turning around failing hotels and then off to the next challenge. We had even purchased a small home in Tucson, Arizona, that would serve as a base so that we always had a place to come home to between assignments.

Our journey in life would take a U-turn at this point, but we did not realize the full scope of this drastic change of direction until after a few years had passed. With Kyler's diagnosis we decided to put my career on hold for a couple of years. From the beginning of Kyler's struggles we seemed to run into just the right person at just the right time with regard to doctors, therapists, interventionists, trainers, teachers, state aides, etc.. If Kyler needed a service, everything seemed to fall into place just as we/he needed it. I knew that if I took a job overseas or across the country these opportunities may not be available for my son, so I decided to sit tight and see how things worked out. The couple of years turned into over a decade, and my professional hopes and dreams would just have to evolve into something different. NO REGRETS HERE!!! Things have not turned out as I had planned, but I have chosen to be grateful for lessons learned, friends made, and my personal journey of discovery.

There is no magic bullet to make everything better or easier on this journey, at least not yet. In fact it seems the more doctors and scientists learn about autism the more they find that there are many different ways/theories on how to deal with its effects and symptoms. It seems no two autistic children are alike. They all have different deficiencies, different areas of difficulty, and in some cases instances of incredible gifts.

I am a father faced with an unknown future and unique circumstances. I am part of a group of fathers that was once a very exclusive club, but is now adding members at an alarming rate. I can view this as a glass half-full or as a glass half-empty life-long proposition. I have decided to look at it as a glass filled to the top with opportunities while on an unusual journey.

In my opinion this is not a case of, "It takes a village to raise a child." Instead, "It takes loving parents with a plan, a lot of professional help, and an open-mind regarding one's core beliefs to raise an autistic child."

Some years ago I was discussing the unique perspective from a father's point of view of having an autistic child with Paula and Noelle, my sons' occupational therapists. As I was expressing these thoughts, feelings, and emotions, (which I assume all fathers must deal with) Paula made an observation I had not considered. She stated that there have been many books written about autism and from many different perspectives. Some are from the clinical point of view; some focus on the many different treatment therapies; some chronicle the path parents have taken to help free their child from a life of darkness and isolation; some recommend diets; many are about the causes of autism; and the list goes on.

With the prevalence of autism now at 1 in 68 (CDC 2014) children born in the United States, one approach Paula mentioned that she has yet to see is how this condition is dealt with from a father's point of view. Paula asked me, "How have you dealt with it as a father? How have you managed to keep your marriage together? How have you faced the difficulties you feel as a father in having a special needs child? Why do you seem to be handling it better then most of the fathers I see?" I considered these questions for some time and was unable to come up with a simple answer. Just saying it was because I loved my wife and children unconditionally would not tell the story. It would not be an honest answer. It would not demonstrate the pain, frustration, and loneliness that every father of a special needs child must endure on his own journey through his child's affliction. The personal pain I face almost daily when I hear of the mental and physical suffering my boys must endure every day can at times be so excruciating that I feel it on a personal, mental, and physical level. I looked deep inside myself to try and understand how I had arrived at this point. How have I survived the often raging emotions, sleepless nights, self denial, frustrations, and soul wrenching pain that comes with learning yours is a special needs offspring?

I have written these words to give voice to the fathers of these children. As a father, how do you explain to *your* father, mother, grandparent, aunt, uncle, cousin, niece, best friend, or any other person you have a relationship with, about your experience? The answer is not simple. How does one chronicle a lifetime of experiences and emotions into a few sentences or a ten-minute conversation? I have tried to explain, teach, and express to others my thoughts and experiences on countless occasions. What I have learned is that it cannot be done and thus the reason for my writing this book. We all must carry our own crosses in life, and unless we walk a mile in someone else's shoes, we can never truly understand what others are going through. Raising a special needs child can be a lifetime challenge for the parents, a lifetime of internal pain that will never be fully extinguished. Each father's journey will be different; every father's pain and burdens will be unique. Unfortunately they will be markedly different than that of a parent of a "normal" child. Though parents will worry about their children for the rest of their lives, the odds are those parents will not have to care for their child the rest of his/her life. The worries about their children will not consume them every day in a manner that can be understood only by another parent of a special needs child. This book is not a pity-party. I would not trade my boys for anything, but it is a glimpse into the private soul of a man who worries every day about the journey of life that must be endured by his very special boys.

INTRODUCTION

"You cannot control the looks, the stares, the judging
from people at the mall or at the store when you have
your child out. You know they're thinking to themselves,
'Hey, why can't they control their child?' The constant
and visual judgment from other people can often be
almost unbearable."

The Race
by D. H. Groberg

"Quit! Give up! You're Beaten!"
They shout at me and plead.
"There's just too much against you now
This time you can't succeed."

And as I start to hang my head in front of failure's face,
My downward fall is broken by the memory of a race.
And hope refills my weakened will as I recall that scene;
For just the thought of that short race rejuvenates my being.

A children's race— young boys, young men—how I remember well.
Excitement sure! But also fear; it wasn't hard to tell.

They all lined up so full of hope, each thought to win that race
Or tie for first, or if not that, at least take second place.
And fathers watched from off the side, each cheering for his son.
And each boy hoped to show his dad that he would be the one.

The whistle blew and off they went, young hearts and hopes afire.
To win and be the hero there was each young boy's desire.
And one boy in particular, whose dad was in the crowd,
Was running near the lead and thought: "My dad will be so proud!"

But as they sped down the field across a shallow dip,
The little boy who thought to win, lost his step and slipped.
Trying hard to catch himself, his hands flew out to brace,
But mid the laughter of the crowd, he fell flat on his face.

So down he fell and with him hope, he couldn't win it now—
Embarrassed, sad, he only wished to disappear somehow.

But as he fell his dad stood up and showed his anxious face,
Which to the boy so clearly said, "Get up and win the race."

He quickly rose, no damage done, behind a bit that's all—
And ran with all his mind and might to make up for his fall.
So anxious to restore himself, to catch up and to win—
His mind went faster than his legs. He slipped and fell again!

He wished then he had quit before, with only one disgrace.
"I'm hopeless as a runner now; I shouldn't try to race."
But in the laughing crowd he searched and found his father's face;
That steady look that said again: "Get up and win the race!"

So he jumped up to try again, ten yards behind the last—
"If I'm to gain those yards," he thought, "I've got to move real fast."
Exerting everything he had, he regained eight or ten,
But trying so hard to catch the lead, he slipped and fell again!

Defeat! He lay there silently. A tear dropped from his eye—
"There's no sense running anymore; three strikes: I'm out! Why try?"
The will to rise had disappeared; all hope had fled away;

So far behind, so error prone; A loser all the way.
"I've lost, so what's the use?" he thought. "I'll live with my disgrace."

But then he thought about his dad, who soon he'd have to face.
"Get up," an echo sounded low, "Get up and take your place;
You were not meant for failure here. Get up and win the race."
"With borrowed will get up," it said, "You haven't lost at all.
For winning is no more than this: To rise each time you fall."

So, up he rose to run once more, and with a new commit
He resolved that Win or Lose, at least he wouldn't quit.
So far behind the others now; the most he'd ever been—
Still he gave it all he had and ran as though to win.

Three times he'd fallen, stumbling; three times he rose again;
Too far behind to hope to win, he still ran to the end.
They cheered the winning runner as he crossed the line first place.
Head high, and proud and happy, no falling, no disgrace.

But when the fallen youngster crossed the line last place,
The crowd gave him the greater cheer, for finishing the race.
And even though he came in last, with head bowed low, unproud,
You would have thought he'd won the race to listen to the crowd.

And to his dad he sadly said, "I didn't do too well."
"To me, you won," his father said. "You rose each time you fell."
And now when things seem dark and hard and difficult to face,
The memory of that little boy helps me in my race.

For all of life is like that race, with ups and downs and all.
And all you have to do to win, is rise each time you fall.

(*The Race* has been printed here in its entirety by request and with permission of the author. Groberg, D.H. *The Race: Life's Greatest Lesson*. New York: Warner Faith. 2004. Print.)

I heard this poem and was brought to tears as I considered my boy's lives and how difficult life will be for them. My sons will fall almost every time they try anything new, and I have to teach them to get up every time without the fanfare or motivation of winning. But what about me? I asked the person whom I had heard recite this poem if he could provide me with a copy. As I read it over a few times, I came to apply it to my own situation but in a different context. My boys don't feel the need to win a race or get any real excitement from the thrill of victory; they're just not wired that way. In fact, a cheering crowd makes them very anxious and uncomfortable, but *I am* wired that way. *I am* wired to win.

In my case, this poem speaks more to how I'm dealing with my sons, and how I'm competing in the race, and how I must continue to get up and finish the race. I am the father. It is my job to get up and support them every time they fail. It is also my job to step up and overcome my own weaknesses and insecurities. Every time I feel discouraged or sad for my boys, I have to remind myself to be strong for them and learn how to help them succeed in their lives. Every time I hear other people criticize or hurt my children, I know it is because of their ignorance about ASD (Autism Spectrum Disorder) and ADHD (Attention Deficit Hyperactivity Disorder), but I honestly feel as though I am taking a physical blow. Every time I am faced with one of my fallen dreams in regard to my sons, and I am knocked to my knees in pain and despair, I have to listen to that voice within me saying, "Get up and win the race!"

In this book you will read about my two autistic sons, Kyler and Koleden. They are both on the autistic spectrum and similar in many ways; however, they are also extremely different from each other. It seems I learn something new about my boys everyday. Just when I think I understand them and understand their disability, a new characteristic or challenge emerges. I have had the fortunate opportunity of meeting with a number of incredible specialists over the years, and slowly I have come to understand a little of what makes my boys tick. After spending two entire days testing and evaluating Kyler, a top neuropsychologist specializing in autism explained to me how Kyler and most autistic children learn. He basically said that autistic kid's minds have multiple file boxes. Unlike normal kids who have the one file box and can cross reference information from one file card to another, autistic children cannot do that. They have to write a new file card for every single action and possibility. They cannot transfer knowledge from one situation to a similar one. They cannot reason that if this worked well for one thing or situation it should work for similar situations quite well. So everything learned must be taught in exacting steps. There can be no assumptions of understanding made, as all teaching must be done step by step with lots of repetition. This makes teaching them difficult and very frustrating for the average person and/or parents, but let me assure you autistic children can be taught with an incredible amount of patience and repetition.

Kyler was born with autism and he is my oldest son. He was also diagnosed with ADHD, Tourette Syndrome, and depression. We caught his problems early and started intense therapy of over 40 hours a week by the time he was three. He had this intensive intervention therapy until the age of eight and then we reduced it to 15 hours a week until the age of 11. He was taught how to do everything—playing with toys, potty training, using a fork, reading facial expressions, talking on the phone, and what to say when he met someone new. He had to be taught everything. He really is a miracle child. We followed what the professionals told us to do to the letter. My wife quit work so that she could do and coordinate all the therapy he needed. He has always been sensory needy and has craved heavy movement in order to keep his system in alignment. Even now after all this therapy and after all the miraculous improvements Kyler has made, he does not comprehend very much. He truly only grasps about 25% of what is spoken. This is especially true when he is part of a group listening to them speak. He often will hear a joke and laugh when everyone else laughs, but will then privately/quietly turn to me and ask me to explain why everyone thought what was said was funny. Even after my explanation he often will say "Dad, I don't get it." He will seldom or never do this with anyone else except his mother or sister. He uses pictures and body language to grasp what people are saying, and this fakes out the casual observer sufficiently. However, if you ask him direct questions to ascertain his comprehension, not yes and no questions, you will quickly come to understand his lack of understanding. He can have a bad temper. He likes to hit his head on the wall or the floor or with his hands. He can be impossible to reason with at these times. He can be fine one second and injure his brother the next without a blink. He has difficulty considering the consequences for his actions, especially if those actions are new and untried. He has few friends but can understand when people are mean to him or exclude him. He understands he is different and that people do not understand how or why he is different. He has been taught to excuse people's actions, and he tries to have empathy, but really does not know how. We cannot yell at him because he internalizes it. Even if we are doing it for positive reasons, he feels that it is "like a whip, lashing him." It is sad.

The truth of the matter is that Kyler is a really good-looking boy. He has seen a large number of "professionals" in his short life, and every therapist's evaluation starts with, "This is a polite, handsome boy." He does not have any outward features that would indicate he is slow, delayed, or debilitated. At recess he can do all the physical activities like any other kid. He is not going to be the best nor will he be the worst. On the playground he just seems like any other kid. It's only when he tries to communicate or when someone lets him go first after rules are explained that problems arise. Kyler's biggest problem occurs when playing games he does not understand. If he doesn't understand the directions to the game being played he will just try to wing it. Unfortunately that does not always work, and he can frustrate the other participants. Even with quick direction from others, he usually does not know what to do. He can be taught how to participate, but it takes time and patience, which is often in short supply in situations like this. He idolizes me and loves me unconditionally.

Koleden was diagnosed with late onset autism. For his first five years he seemed to be my wife's "gift" after struggling with Kyler. Everything changed after we got his inoculations (we do not blame his inoculation per se but we do know that this was when his digression began.) He now has a diagnosis of classically high-functioning autism. He is also diagnosed with depression, ADD, self-multilation, and Tourettes. He was provided with none of the help that his older brother received. He likes to be by himself. He is very good in math and engineering. He loves computer time and playing on the X-box and mobile gaming devices. **He has no friends**. He has no social skills and does not understand social cues. He is obsessive and compulsive in many areas. He is addicted to tattling on others and enforcing rules. He gets emotional easily, and when this happens he shuts down, becoming rigidly unreasonable. At these times, we cannot reach him, as he mentally withdraws into his own personal space. However he can be the most loving of my children. He can be the most empathetic of all of them. I have worked extremely hard over the last few years to force Koleden to accept physical hugs and closeness. He likes to sleep in a nylon sleeve/cocoon that is made for a child under 5' and 100 lbs., even though he is much larger than that. Now he will sit next to me and cuddle; okay he will sit close to me and let me hold him. It is fun to cuddle my 152 lb, 5'6", 13 year old. He is so funny. He is so literal that I have to be careful what I say. He is sensitive to noise and large crowded spaces. He does not do well with chaos. We have often received disapproving stares when we have had to cover his ears or allow him to use headphones in concerts, recitals, or performances by our daughters. He self-mutilates when he is upset or frustrated. He doesn't even realize he is doing it. He will literally chew his fingers to bloody ends and his eyes will be vacant. He will be in his own world trying to escape whatever it is that is overwhelming his system. He finds smelling his fingers calming; however, this is not a characteristic that junior high kids find attractive, and this causes him to be the center of some cruel bullying. He is awkward due to a birth defect of his right leg. It causes him to have bad balance and it hurts him to run or walk for any length of time. Again, this is not popular among his age group. He definitely does not fit into a group.

These are my sons in a nutshell. You will learn more as you read this book. I love them for who they are. I am so blessed to have them. The race we run everyday reminds me that it is I who need to get up every time I fall. It is I who needs to hold my head up high and learn from my boys. To win the race I just have to keep living each day and trying to be a better dad.

HAVE YOU EVER?

By Tassy Tomlin

Have you ever wished you could hold and receive affection from your child? Have you ever wished your child would look at you the fifth, sixth or seventh time you called his name? Have you ever wished he would call you [daddy, dad, or da]? Have you ever wished your 2- year old would tell you NO? Have you ever pointed to 8 different boxes of cereal to see which box he wants because he can't tell you? Have you ever wondered why the things he does say, he says over and over? Have you ever been blessed with a smile from ear to ear because you understood what he meant the first time he tried to tell you something? Have you ever let him eat cereal all day long because that's almost all he will eat? Have you fixed pizza ten or more times a week because he'll eat that too? Have you ever washed that special plate and bowl 2 or 3 times a day because he has to eat off of them? Have you ever had to get up from the table twice in one sitting to wash his precious hands because they got dirty and he won't eat until they're clean? Have you ever let your child wear the same shirt for 3 days in a row, thanking God at least he's wearing clothes today? Have you ever taken his shoes off and put them back on 6 or 7 times, until they feel just right? Have you ever let him wear those shoes to bed, night after night?

Have you ever wondered why he tiptoed all day long and could never sit still? Have you ever let him wear a sock hat all day and to bed because the pressure makes him feel a little better and covering his ears muffles a fraction of the night time noise? Have you ever wondered why out of all the toys he has to play with, he stares at the wheels of the car he rolls back and forth? Have you ever wondered why he doesn't play? Have you ever had to draw the Wal-Mart star or spark twenty or more times a day? Have you ever had to ask the manager at Wal-Mart for a sign, so you wouldn't have to draw it all day? Have you ever seen the joy on your child's face to have that sign? Have you ever had to ask the manager at a restaurant if you could let him sneak a quick look at the kitchen before he'd sit down to eat? Have you ever had to get up and leave a restaurant as soon as your food hits the table? Have you been in the checkout line, with a cart full of groceries, when a major meltdown hits? Have you ever watched people stare at you and your child like you both have the plague? Have you then had to hold your head high and bite your lip for the sake of your child? Have you ever had to convince your pediatrician that something's just not right? Have you ever had to sit through hours of intensive evaluations, scared of the unknown? Have you ever received the diagnosis of Autism for your child?

CHAPTER ONE

THE CALLS

*"When you get the diagnosis you ask what does it mean,
but there are no clear answers."*

*"I once heard this quote from a motivational speaker that
really hit home: 'Come what may and love it.' I felt these
words were said directly to me on how to cope with my
boys and the life I live."*

Every so often I get calls from friends or relatives asking if they can give my number to someone who may have or who has an autistic, ADD, ADHD, or some other developmental disordered child. They want to hear our story. Of course I gladly take these calls. I generally plan on a couple of hours for them. I'll sit alone in the living room, get comfortable, and dial the person. Usually it's the mom who calls and it always starts the same. After the introductions we start talking about the behaviors and tests they have had, the professionals they have seen up until now. I tell them that I'm not a doctor or a trained professional but just a dad who would be glad to share a little of what I have learned through the years. What they want to hear and what I tell them never seems to be in sync. What people want to hear is that everything is going to be okay. A few visits to the doctor and some therapy and wham-o everything is fixed and their child is better and they're off on their merry way, back on track with a regular life. My wife and I often ask ourselves if we are just too honest, sometimes brutally so, but we were in those shoes once and found almost no answers out there, and we know what it is like to attack this thing without a clue as to where we are going or how we are going to get there.

After listening to the symptoms, I ask them some basic questions. Does your child mutilate his food? Does he hit his head over and over? Does he scream non-stop? Does he constantly jump off the furniture? Does he have any language problems? How many different kinds of food will he eat? Does he line objects up in perfect rows? Does he obsess over anything? Does he socialize or play well with other children? As the list grows, the parent begins to realize that we understand what they are going through.

My first suggestion is to get a proper diagnosis from a qualified neurologist or psychiatrist. Of course I am not qualified to provide any kind of diagnosis. Then the conversation invariably turns to what their life is going to be like in the near, short term future as they try to find out where their child is on the ASD spectrum, if they are even on it at all. Some kids just have more energy than others and what they may fear as autism is really just a bit of extra spunk that will abate with time. However, if parents have suspicions something is wrong, I always tell them they should have their child see an appropriate doctor as soon as possible.

Because parents want to hear about our experiences, I talk about our oldest son and his early intervention and how studies have proven that the earlier you can catch autism the better. I discuss a little about my first son who was born with classic autistic symptoms that were evident early, then I share our experience with our second son who was late onset and how they are different. I review how no two autistic children are the same. I relate our experiences with the different state agencies in Arizona and how they have helped us. I talk about the statistics of how pervasive autism is now compared to just 15-20 yrs ago. I give them a few websites where they can go for information (autismspeaks.org, autismcenter.org, familiesforautism.org). I also let them know about how loving our boys are and also what a wonderful blessing they are in our lives, and that we would not change them for anything.

The most common question I get from these calls or interviews is, "Is the autism diagnosis going to change our life and how?" This is the question that people struggle with. The answer is that it all depends on you and if you love your child unconditionally, because if you do, this is where the rubber hits the road. The answer will be "Of course, tremendously." Your life will never be the same. You will never fit into the mold of "normal" again. Your life is going to go off into directions you never thought possible or even considered. You will be scared and at many times unsure what to do for your child. If you have other children, their lives will also change forever. They will face many challenges that you will need to face with them. You will need to become a tower of strength and knowledge. You will need to learn all you can about your child's diagnosis. As a parent you will also be learning about the mind and learning ability of your special needs child, and you will slowly learn how your child's learning occurs.

No two Autistic or Asperger's Syndrome children are the same, and though many can learn and be taught, it is often in a different manner than you are accustomed to or familiar with. They all have social issues and some odd or repetitive behaviors. While in public, these odd behaviors will make you and your child seem peculiar to other people. You will need to become your child's advocate in your family, school, community, and even church. You will need to support your other children and let them know they are not forgotten in the craziness that will occur as you develop a plan for the treatment of your autistic child. So, yes, your life will change immensely. Sometimes you will think only of the total change of life this diagnosis will impose on the family, but if you try, you can come to appreciate the new perspective your child will give you on life in general.

As parents, your lives will never be the same and you will need to adjust and accept. People do not want to hear that their lives must change. They do not want their other children to be affected. They do not want professionals telling them that they are parenting incorrectly for a special needs child. They struggle with the concept that developmental experts have a better understanding of what's best for their child. Many experts do in fact have a great understanding of how to help you develop desired behaviors for your special needs child. The parents we talk to are always surprised when we say these things, but they need to be said. Hopefully it will ease their transition into the treatment for their child. In other words, they need to get out of the way and let the professionals do their jobs to help them on their new and unexpected journey through life.

CHAPTER TWO

WHY DON'T KIDS COME WITH MANUALS?

*"There is no playbook. There is no textbook.
There are no directions. There is no one telling you
what the future will hold."*

*"You ask over and over what will happen
when he grows up?
There is no answer. No one knows."*

This is an age old question that has been posed and written about by thousands upon thousands of authors in almost every language. But our own personal upbringing as well as our observations of others tend to be our real guide. Some people read books and do their best to follow them. Some people go to classes and educate themselves with higher learning. Lastly, some just wing it. Whatever your method, I'm here to tell you when dealing with your autistic child, **in the beginning you do not know best!** I'm not actually sure anyone does, but there have been some incredible advancements in the treatment of these very special kids. And from our experience the person who needs the most treatment and the most change is YOU THE PARENT. Remember this is not about you; it's about you as the parent of an autistic child. You are going to be the one who will have the most impact on that child's life. In many cases he/she will live with you for the rest of your life.

When Kyler, my first son, was diagnosed with autism, there were not a lot of great books that explained what was going on and what autism meant in terms that parents could understand. We did read a few books on the topic; however, they always attacked it from a clinical point of view, with few actual stories of individuals and their families. Most of it was so clinically written it went way over my head.

We were guided to a book, _A Parent's Guide to Asperger Syndrome & High-Functioning Autism_, by Sally Ozonoff, Geraldine Dawson, and James McPartland, that was extremely helpful. It provided the following criteria that was used in the diagnosis for our son. We were able to actually see where his deficiencies were. It provided us with a simple-to-understand guideline of where we were and a limited idea of where we might be going.

The **DSM-IV Criteria for Autistic Disorder (as used for our sons, 1996 & 2004):** [There is now DSM-V that is significantly different from the these criteria.] To be diagnosed with autistic disorder, Kyler, our oldest son, had to have difficulty in three areas: social relating, communication, and behaviors & interests. He also had to display at least 6 of the 12 symptoms below. He had to experience at least two of the symptoms in the "reciprocal social interaction" domain, at least one symptom in the "communication" domain, and at least one symptom in the "restricted, repetitive behaviors" section. At least one difficulty must have been present before the age of three.

The **DSM-IV Criteria for Autistic Disorder** is shown on the following pages.

DSM-IV Symptoms (must have 6 of 12) Examples

DEFICITS IN RECIPROCAL SOCIAL INTERACTION
(At least 2 symptoms)

1a. Difficulty using nonverbal behaviors to regulate social interaction
   - Trouble looking other in the eye
   - Little use of gestures while speaking
   - Few or unusual facial expressions
   - Trouble knowing how close to stand to others
   - Unusual intonation or voice quality

1b. Failure to develop age-appropriate peer relationships
   - Few or no friends
   - Relationships only with those much older or younger than the child or with family
   - Relationships based primarily on special interests
   - Trouble interacting in groups and following cooperative rules of games

1c. Little sharing of pleasure
   - Enjoys favorite activities, TV shows, toys alone, without trying to involve other people
   - Does not try to call other's attention to activities, interests, or accomplishments
   - Little interest in or reaction to praise

1d. Lack of social or emotional reciprocity
   - Does not respond to others: "appears deaf"
   - Not aware of others: "oblivious" to their existence
   - Strongly prefers solitary activities
   - Does not notice when others are hurt or upset; does not offer comfort

DEFICITS IN COMMUNICATION (At least 1 symptom)

2a. Delay in or total lack of development of language
–No use of words to communicate by age 2
–No simple phrases (for example, "More milk") by age 3
–After speech develops, immature grammar or repeated errors

2b. Difficulty holding conversations
–Has trouble knowing how to start, keep going, and/or end a
conversation
–Little back-and-forth; may talk on and on in a monologue
–Fails to respond to the comments of others; responds only to
direct questions
–Difficulty talking about topics not of special interest

2c. Unusual or repetitive language
–Repeating what others say to them (echolalia)
–Repeating from videos, books, or commercials at inappropriate
times or out of context
–Using words or phrases that the child has made up or that have
special meaning only to him/her
–Overly formal, pedantic style of speaking (sounds like "a little
professor")

2d. Play that is not appropriate for development level
–Little acting-out scenario with toys
–Rarely pretends an object is something else (for example, a
banana is a telephone)
–Prefers to use toys in a concrete manner (for example, building
with blocks, arranging dollhouse furniture) rather than
pretending with them
–When young, little interest in social games like peekaboo,
ring-around-the Rosie

RESTRICTED, REPETITIVE BEHAVIORS, INTERESTS OR ACTIVITIES (At least 1 symptom)

3a. Interests that are narrow in focus, overly intense, and/or unusual
–Very strong focus on particular topics to the exclusion of other topics
–Difficulty "letting go" of special topics or activities
–Interference with other activities (for example delays eating or toileting due to focus on activity)
–Interest in topics that are unusual for age (sprinkler systems, movie ratings, astrophysics, radio station call letters)
–Excellent memory for details of special interests

3b. Unreasonable insistence on sameness and following familiar routines
–Wants to perform certain activities in an exact order (for example, close car doors in specific order)
–Easily upset by minor changes in routine (for example, taking a different route home from school)
–Need for advanced warning of any changes
–Becomes highly anxious and upset if routines or rituals not followed

3c. Repetitive motor mannerisms
–Flapping hands when excited or upset
–Flicking fingers in front of eyes
–Odd hand postures or other hand movements
–Spinning or rocking for long periods of time
–Walking and/or running on tiptoe

3d. Preoccupation with parts of objects
–Uses objects in unusual ways (for example, flicks doll's eyes, repeatedly opens and closes doors on a toy car), rather than as intended

–Interest in sensory qualities of object (for example, like to sniff objects or look at them closely)
–Likes objects that move (for example, fans, running water, spinning wheels)
–Attachment to unusual objects (for example, orange peel, string)

Ozonoff, Sally, & Dawson, Geraldine, & McPartland, James. *A Parent's Guide to Asperger Syndrome & High-Functioning Autism.* New York: Guilford Press. (pp 27-28), 2002.

For Kyler these were easy for us to see because there was no question he was born with autism. For my second son, Koleden, it was much harder because he was late onset, and we had been in denial of acknowledging any of the weird quirks he had developed until after his diagnosis. We actually used it as a checklist with my wife making notes in the book where they did apply to my boys.

By using the above criteria my son Kyler exhibited 11 of the 12 symptoms. Of the 49 examples within those symptoms he displayed 40 of them. This was staggering. Koleden, my second son, exhibited 12 of the 12 symptoms and 32 of the 49 examples.

There was not going to be any manual to guide us on how to handle and teach my boys who were so different from the norm. All my wife and I could do was educate ourselves and turn unequivocally to the experts.

CHAPTER THREE
Our Parenting Philosophy

"A health teacher once told my daughter that autism was caused by moms that just watched television, smoked, drank, and ate bon-bons—the refrigerator mom. That really set me off."

To understand how we decided to parent, one must understand where we came from. My wife, Dana, came from a white, middle-class home. There was no real corporal punishment. She could count the times she was spanked. Punishment was done by both parents and usually through behavior modification. Both her parents were teachers and highly educated. Her mother taught child development at the University of Arizona and was a very good role model. They expected Dana to graduate from high school with high grades and go on to college to get a bachelor's degree.

My upbringing could not have been more different. I was raised in a fairly strict middle to low-income Hispanic home. Both my mother and my father were born in Mexico, so I am first generation American born. As the oldest of 8 children, I was expected to be a good kid, which was generally true. The expectation was that I would graduate from high school with any grades possible. There was no thought of college. My siblings and I were raised to do as we were told, for not doing so would get us some form of corporal punishment. "Children were to be seen and not heard." As my father often said, "Do as I say, not as I do."

My mother was the real disciplinarian in the family. Her children often triggered her fairly short temper. Our dad was usually pretty easy-going, but on the rare occasion one of us did something that embarrassed him or his parenting, then we had better watch out. He could get quite physical, and he did knock us older boys around fairly well on a few occasions. I tended not to be much on the receiving end of this, as I was too scared most of the time to do anything wrong. My younger brother (by 11 1/2 months), on the other hand, seemed to fall on the wrong side of things with my dad from time to time. I tried hard to learn from his mistakes. Though not always successful, I did manage to avoid more trouble with my dad than my brother did. As far as my mother was concerned, it was impossible to stay out of her way. Her emotions could flip in an instant and then she would go from happy mom to raving mad, and any implement was fair game to use for hitting us. Usually it was a wooden spoon or a shoe, but it could be a number of other household items. Again, my younger brother got more than his fair share of the negative attention, but I was in no way spared this experience.

So why do I share this sad but true dirty laundry of my generally happy upbringing? Well, our experiences define who we are, and if we can identify these experiences then we have a better chance to redefine who we become. The saying is, "History repeats itself." Well, it was my plan to be a different parent, as far as a disciplinarian, than my parents. So prior to marriage, and prior to having kids, my wife and I spent many days and nights discussing how we were going to parent. We consciously watched what and how other parents did things. We asked questions of others' parenting philosophies, matching that to how we saw their children behaving. We read books on parenting, watched movies, and just observed as much as we could from others. We made it a study of sorts. We waited five years to have kids. We wanted to be the best parents we could be. Isn't that the aim of all parents? We want to be better than our parents were and raise kids who are a credit to themselves and productive members of society. So here are a few of the guidelines we set for ourselves prior to having children. I know many people will disagree with our methods, but they are what we came up with after much thought and consideration, taking into account our diverse backgrounds.

-Consistency in what we expected: For example we used the 1,2,3 method of counting to allow the child to change his/her actions. We could count out loud or we could use our fingers. Either choice was fine. The consistency was that if we started to count we <u>always</u> had to follow through on our expectations, no exception, no stretching out the counting. If we got to three, action was required. Sometimes that meant getting up from watching a movie or stopping a project to correct an action by the child, or even stopping the car, but consistency was the key. Don't start counting unless you were going to follow through.

-Corporal punishment was allowed but with caveats. Striking was only on the hands or butt, never more then 3 times, never with an instrument, only with the hand, and never while angry. A rare pop on the mouth was allowed, but no slapping. Belt spankings (3 swats max) were also allowed but only after consultation between parents and for only the most grievous offenses, i.e. stealing or intentionally hurting another person. This would always be preceded and followed by a discussion with the child why this was being done and reviewing what they did wrong as well as hugs and kisses. It was the rare exception that this was done, but as my children will attest—it did happen.

Brenna, our first child and daughter, lulled us into thinking that our parenting skills were just so well conceived that we had it all figured out. She was the model baby and toddler. Everyone loved her. She was never a problem. People remarked all the time that her behavior was amazing. She was polite and respectful and a joy to be around.

We were ready to have another child. Since my brother and I are only 11 1/2 months apart, I wanted to have our next child quickly. My brother and I were best friends while growing up, and I wanted that for my kids. Luckily my wife agreed. So 17 months after Brenna was born, our son came into the world, Kyler.

CHAPTER FOUR

Kyler's Birth

"I don't want my son to be a simpleton!"

My wife's pregnancy was as normal as pregnancies can be except that she was 10 days overdue. There was a concern that the baby would get too big to safely have him vaginally, so she was scheduled to be induced. The day started early as we had an hour drive to the hospital and we were scheduled to be there at 7:00 a.m. We arrived at the hospital and were quickly admitted. My wife had started having labor pains sometime in the early morning. Once admitted to a birthing room, Dana did not tell the nurse she was having pains. She wanted to make sure she was given pitocin to ensure the birth would be forthcoming. The reason for this was that our first child, Brenna, did not come easily. Labor and delivery for Brenna lasted over 50 hours with prodromal labor. Dana had endured labor pains every 3 minutes or less for over two days. She did not want to go through that again. She was fearful of another lengthy exhausting labor.

After having the pitocin started and gel applied to the appropriate areas, the nurse left us, expecting labor would be shortly starting. The nurse came back later and placed some monitoring devices on Dana to track her contractions and vital signs. Once the nurse had everything in place, she noted that Dana was in the beginnings of labor. She checked Dana's birthing condition but determined it was still early in the labor process. The nurse came in to do her hourly checks and my wife went from 10% effaced to 100% in just a few minutes. It was time!!

We ran into a small snag at this point. The doctor was nowhere to be found and Kyler was coming. So the nurse checked Dana again and there he was, crowned. What happened next was and is still a concern. The nurse told her to stop pushing. We needed to wait for the doctor to arrive. I wanted to get angry, demand that they help my wife deliver the baby, but I acquiesced to the professionals. Who was I to tell them what to do? We waited for 35 minutes with Kyler crowned and ready to come. Dana struggled to keep him in. They kept telling her to blow a feather so she wouldn't push him out. Once the doctor arrived she didn't even have time to slip on a gown. She put on her gloves, had a seat in the rolling chair, and one push later he was out. To this day we wonder if this was the right decision, allowing him to stay in the crowned position for so long. We try not to dwell on that thought. We can't change it.

Kyler came out angry, so there was no need to tap him on the butt. He spent most of his first day in the world crying at the top of his lungs. Even the nurses commented that he was an angry baby. We do not know what, if any, bearing this extended birthing procedure and holding period had on his condition, but it is part of his story and will always be a question mark. His head sustained pressure on his brain for 35 minutes. It will always be an unknown factor. His APGAR (Appearance, Pulse, Grimace, Activity, Respiration) scores were normal across the board.

CHAPTER FIVE

A DAD'S DREAM

*"Will he ever learn to walk? Will he ever learn to speak?
Will he ever learn to eat? Will he ever go to school? Will
he ever have friends? Will he ever go to dances? Will he
ever play on an athletic team? Will he ever be popular in
school? Will he ever have a girlfriend? Will he ever finish
high school? When will he graduate? Will he go to college?
Will he be able to hold down a job? Will he be able to get
married? Will he be able to have children? Will he be able
to support himself? Will he, Will he,
Will he...."*

My son's resume of athletic progenitors is pretty impressive. Great-grandmother played basketball for the Mexican National team. Grandfather was a 3-Sport Letterman at the University of Arizona and is a member of every Sports' Hall of Fame in Arizona as both a player and a coach. An uncle represented the United States at the Para-Olympics on the United States Basketball team and was named the United States Team MVP. An aunt was the top ranked professional female boxer in the world in the flyweight division. Add to that a cousin who is an Olympic Silver Medalist in swimming. Do you see where this is going?

As a father I also brought a little to the table in the athletic arena. I was an above average athlete in high school. I played 3 sports and was named to every Arizona All-Everything team in baseball my junior and senior years. The baseball teams I played on always played in the High School State Championship game. I was good enough to go to college on a baseball scholarship and have a great experience. I had the chance to play softball on a USA Select National team that played a tournament in the Bahamas. I met my wife right after she returned from her first year attending BYU-Hawaii where she was an Academic All-American on the National Championship collegiate volleyball team. She was also a 3-sport varsity letterman 3 years in high school and an Arizona State Champion in basketball with the only undefeated season for the huge 5A division in Arizona.

Bill Cosby, the incredibly talented comedian, does a very funny skit in "Bill Cosby Himself," regarding his son and the dreams of his child's greatness on the gridiron. Every athletic father has these feelings when he finds out he is going to have a son, someone to carry on the family name and do it with athletic greatness. There was a clean slate for his offspring to etch the name with accomplishments. With his mom's brains and both of our athletic backgrounds, the world was his for the taking—junior sports then on to high school and college. The world had no limit for my new son.

That was my dream! Why shouldn't it be? I was the dad who would have a great athlete with the smarts to go with it. Maybe he would be popular, well-liked, have lots of friends, be a leader of people, get good grades, be a college graduate, All-State athlete, Academic All-American, father of my grandchildren, fishing buddy, golf partner, and all around great friend. My dreams were about to be crushed, and though it took me a long time to come to this realization, I eventually did.

CHAPTER SIX

REALITY HITS

"I worry that he might do something horrific someday to hurt other people, not understanding what his actions are or what the consequences could be."

Kyler never liked to lie down flat from the moment we brought him home. We quickly learned he loved being in his car seat and the tighter strapped in the better. We would get home from anywhere and if he was asleep in his car seat, we left him in it. He would stay there asleep on the living room floor for hours. For the first 11 months of his life he would sleep only sitting up in his car seat. One of his favorite activities was to look at his hands and open and close them in front of his face for hours. He loved to watch Disney cartoons in that seat. As an infant, sometimes while watching Disney cartoons was the only time he would stop opening and closing his fists. He would go through phases of which movies he liked to watch, but this was almost always done from the car seat, truly his favorite place. He also liked his swing where he could sit up and watch the TV. When we told the pediatrician about these strange behaviors, we were told not to worry. Autism was so rare at this time that it was not on a pediatrician's radar or closely monitored.

As I mentioned, Kyler showed that all-so-typical autistic trait of playing/shaking his hands in his face for long periods of time. He kept himself quite occupied with this pastime. Often even while watching his favorite cartoon he would do this; at dinner he would do this; or just riding in the car he would do this. I think you get the picture. He was also a screamer. During his infant and toddler years he never developed sounds or words that meant anything. We constantly brought this up at check-ups, but the doctor always told us that he was a boy, a second child, and the behavior was normal.

My wife finally put her foot down when Kyler was 15 months old and there were no words at all, only screaming. She demanded that the doctor give her the referral to see a speech specialist. Our insurance would not pay for speech therapy until an auditory test was done, so we were sent to an Ears, Nose, and Throat (ENT) specialist. At first we were told that his severe speech delay (or non-verbalness) was due to his constant ear infections. The doctor told us that his hearing was like trying to hear and speak while 5-feet under water. We were told that if we got tubes for his ears, his speech would start developing. I hated the thought of having our son go into sedated surgery at such a young age, but we listened to the doctor, which became a prevailing theme for most of our son's life. With the procedure complete, our question for the doctor was how long before we should see improvement in his speech? The reply was that in the next 4-6 weeks he should start using some words. He would be delayed for a while but he would catch up quickly.

As a few months passed we did not see any improvement in our son. There were the return visits to the ENT doctor to check if the tubes had fallen out, but they were still in and the opinion was that he was a second child and a boy and that he would be fine. However, my son wasn't fine and there was still no improvement. We were finally granted a referral for speech therapy. Our insurance would pay for 24 visits a year. Visits to doctors and specialists began very early on in my son's pre-diagnosis stage. So began the searching for answers, the checklist which would one day lead to his diagnosis.

At this point in his life Kyler had been doing a few things that were just plain weird, and some things that were annoying. We learned much later that all these actions are fairly common with autistic kids: hitting his head, throwing toys, walking aimlessly, screaming, **(and I mean screaming, for hours at the top of his lungs)** while opening and closing his hands! If he wanted something, anything, you knew it by his high pitched, very loud scream. We would try to figure out what he wanted us to get him to calm down, and we were so relieved when we succeeded in making him happy and quiet. As you can imagine, trips out of the house anywhere were stressful. People were always looking at us and wondering why we couldn't control our kid. This was both embarrassing and made me angry that other people were judging me. My wife came home crying one day from a trip to the store because some woman told her she was a bad parent because of how badly her child was behaving. I wanted to go and find that lady and give her a piece of my mind. We stopped taking him out. If my wife had to do some shopping she would leave him with her mother. If we had to go out, we never took him; it just was not worth the embarrassment and looks we got from everyone, everywhere.

Jumping from anything and landing on the floor for hours and hours on end was another must-do for Kyler. This was an annoying activity. I suppose all parents are a bit worried about kids hurting themselves. Well, Kyler was not afraid of anything, most of all heights or the possibility of pain. In fact this boy felt no pain. He would run across the room and jump into the couch at full speed. Of course his sister would join him for this fun, squealing, good time, and she would tire of it after awhile, but not Kyler. He would go for hours. We thought he was going to ruin our new leather couch with this behavior, which of course he did. My wife eventually had to re-fill the back seat cushions a few times because they got so flat. Unlike most toddlers who have a cute little belly, Kyler had 6-pack abs and muscle defined legs. It was amazing.

As he got a little older we were able to get him out of his car seat and into the crib in his room for sleep. He would, of course, scream, then start jumping up and down in his bed. We had a nice crib with an innerspring mattress and a spring support under it. His jumping often went on well past midnight before he went to sleep. Another strange thing he did was to pile all the blankets and pillows on top of him so they created pressure on his body as he slept. He would stick his butt in the air like a beetle and hold his arms and legs in close to his body. Then he was up no later than 5:00 a.m., to start the jumping all over again and off to start another day of blood curdling screams and non-stop jumping. Had it not been for a few movies which he would often mimic the actions to (Mary Poppins and Chitti-Chitti Bang-Bang dance scenes) which he watched so many times the tapes got ruined, my wife's entire day would have been spent keeping him from hurting himself.

Food mutilation and "chimpmunking" was also a favorite pastime of his. Meal time was always interesting. I suppose all kids throw their food, at least all our kids did, but Kyler took it to a new level. Getting him to try foods was quite difficult, okay—impossible. He would first play with it, smashing it in his hands until it was mush. Then he would throw it everywhere or put it all over himself. That meant we needed to feed him, 'cause "He has got to eat." Right? He would chew his food, or so we thought, seem to be full, and refuse more. Then a couple of hours later we would find the last of his meal stored in his cheeks, and he would spit it out, or we would have to dig it out. Of course we caught onto this pretty fast and just resigned ourselves to the fact he was a picky eater. We gave him exactly what he would eat, which was not much. This was annoying to me because I had been raised to eat what was put in front of me, and here was my child not really eating and defying us regarding his diet. This was just not acceptable. I spent many frustrating hours trying to force feed him or go to the other extreme of not feeding him at all and just putting him to bed with no dinner. It seems I would go from one extreme to the other without any real consistency to my behavior. I was getting more and more frustrated with my son, and had it not been for my level headed wife, I honestly do not know how I might have acted or what I may have done to try to teach that kid one way or another.

Milk is always a major concern for little ones. Kyler would drink only Shamrock chocolate milk. He knew by taste and/or texture if it was not Shamrock. We were strapped for cash in those days and Shamrock milk was one of the most expensive brands available in our market. Dana would try mixing the powdered stuff and putting it in the Shamrock bottles, buying the cheaper stuff and putting it in the Shamrock bottle, not showing the bottle at all, but Kyler always, and I mean always knew the difference. He was and still is very sensitive to food texture. He did not like anything crunchy. He liked pancakes but only a certain brand and a certain type of syrup, moist Eggo Waffles, Kraft Mac-n-Cheese but not the Kraft Easy-Mac, beef Top Ramen soup, no vegetables, no fruit except for Gala apples with no skin, and of course he would eat almost any sweets. He definitely did and does have a major sweet tooth.

So that is a snapshot of our early years with Kyler. Many of his actions almost sent me over the edge. If it hadn't been for a well-defined disciplinary plan, I think my temper might have gotten the best of me. Not to say I did not give him a swat for his unruly behavior; I most assuredly did, but it was not very effective. Phil, a friend and also the father of an autistic son, once told me, "You can't beat autism out of a child." I'm glad I learned that lesson kind of early.

It took me a number of years to learn the most important fact about the treatment and hopeful progress we were going to make with Kyler's development. No amount of discipline, scoldings, spankings, deprivations, or any other kinds of punishments were going to help in the development of my son. NONE, NADA, ZILCH. A dog can be treated this way with moderate success, but an autistic child <u>will never</u> reach his/her potential if that is the approach that is taken.

I must also add that a 180 degree approach to the above is equally ineffective. Coddling, spoiling, indulging, pampering, and babying will not garner the desired outcomes, because autism is a neurological disorder not a behavioral disorder.

As I reflect on those times, I just shake my head when I consider my actions, my attitudes, my stubbornness. This is a shame I will carry with me always. I know today I am a better man than I once was, but I will never be able to change my past actions; they are written in stone, but not my future actions. I still have the chance to be better, to do better, and this is my present journey.

CHAPTER SEVEN

THERAPIES BEGIN

"Some say he's just a second child; he'll grow out of it. I wonder, 'What makes you the expert?' If I had followed this advice he'd still be sitting in a corner hitting himself on the head, wearing a diaper, nonverbal, malnutritioned, and an absolute drain on everyone and everything around him."

Kyler had yet to be diagnosed with autism at 19 months. Nina, the young speech therapist we had been referred to, had just 24 visits to work with Kyler, as per our insurance. After the third visit Nina told us there would be little she could do to help us with Kyler's speech. He didn't even know how to play with toys. All he did was throw them: crayons, cars, puzzle pieces, any and all toys presented to him. The only words he had were "Thank you" and that was discernible only to us and Nina. She told us we needed to go to the Arizona Division of Developmental Disability (DDD) and get into the program for some occupational therapy and some more speech. At 24 months we were recommended to an occupational therapist, (OT), Paula. Autism was the furthest thing from our minds as we made that first visit with her. That was the beginning of our journey into the daunting world of autism. Thus began the real struggle.

Paula peppered us with questions about Kyler's development. She was great at asking questions and getting us to provide all the little details about our son without it seeming to be a checklist of milestones to determine Kyler's severity of some form of Development Delayed

Disorder. She did comment that his gross motor skills were highly developed for his age. He actually had muscles in his thighs, and as I mentioned before, he had a 6-pack for abs. There was no baby fat tummy on our 2-year old.

I was resistant to taking Kyler to occupational therapy. I was adamant that nothing could possibly be wrong with him except perhaps a little development delay. My reasoning was that Kyler could hit and throw a ball really well for a small guy. We could play hitting the ball for hours in the back yard. He had great eye-hand coordination. He could accurately throw and even catch a ball from 20 to 30 feet away. Of course he had other issues like needing heavy movement, smashing his food, and never making eye contact, but we all know adults that are like that. To me those weren't important deficiencies. He could play ball and that was all that mattered. He seemed to have great athletic ability, and my dream was about to be fulfilled. Kyler demonstrated excellent big muscle control and had a little body builder's body, with all his muscles rippling. All was as it should be.

I was later to learn that Paula strongly suspected autism as a possible diagnosis. She was just unsure as to how severe. Unfortunately, she was not qualified to give us a diagnosis, so she kept those thoughts to herself. I'm sure it was difficult for a person like Paula to know what life-altering and shattering events would be unfolding for a family in the near future but unable herself to provide the diagnosis. The amazing thing about Paula is that after 25 years of helping these special people, she continues her life-long goal of making a difference regardless of the inner battle she faces every time a new charge comes into her play room.

Our state-assigned interventionist, Gayle, worked with Paula, and they helped where they could in guiding us to to get tests and evaluations, but as they were not qualified to give us a diagnosis, they kept those thoughts to themselves. We did not overly press Paula for her feelings on a possible diagnosis, because we had no idea of the road we were heading down. To tell you the truth, we were not even close to being ready to hear it. We began with what was called a "Kids' Club" that met twice a week. We also had an hour of speech, an hour of occupational therapy, and an hour of sensory integration every week. As per DDD, Kyler was on this broad spectrum of pervasive developmentally delayed treatment across the board. It was at that juncture that my wife and I decided she needed to give up her job of high school teacher/coach so that she could be with Kyler and do whatever we could to help him catch up with his peers and be age-appropriate. It took 6 months of this routine for Paula, Gayle, and the speech therapist, Nancy, finally to convince us to see a pediatric neurologist.

CHAPTER EIGHT

DIAGNOSIS

"I lie awake all night sometimes, wondering what is going to happen to my boys, but no one seems able to give us an answer or idea."

Our first visit to the pediatric neurologist was like a freight train hitting us. However, as time went on we learned that what she shared with us that day was a train in the far distance. Think of standing on a train track at night looking far into the distance to where a train should be coming. You can't hear it, but you know it's coming. You don't have any idea if it is just the one locomotive or a train a mile long. You just know it's coming. Will it stop before it gets to you? You just don't know. So our journey began. At the age of 2 1/2 Kyler was officially diagnosed with autism.

The day we received Kyler's diagnosis is still crystal clear in my mind. It was the day that changed the world around us, and it was truly earth shattering, but to what extent we really had no idea at the time. When I think about that day, it seems so far away, but it plays just like a movie in my mind. We returned home from the 30-minute drive from the neurologist with hardly a word spoken between us. We were both dumbfounded. We did not even know what autism meant. The doctor had tried to give us an example, but we were in too much shock for it to compute. We walked into our bedroom and sat on the edge of the bed just stunned at the news. The flood of emotions that my wife was feeling came out in a tidal wave; she slumped to the floor and started to cry. It was not just tears but huge sobs and pitiful questions. Why did this happen to her? Was she a bad person? Why had God done this to us? What did we do to deserve this? What are we going to do? What does it all mean? I felt so helpless as I reached out to her, unable to comfort her, unable to be the strong man with the answers and solutions. I was not sure what it all meant, but I saw my bride in heart-wrenching pain, and there was very little I could do about it. I did all I could in that situation. I held her and tried to assure her that everything would be okay. We sat there on the floor for what seemed a very long time, with my wife going from crying to sobbing while I held her in my arms. THIS WAS OUR FIRST OFFICIAL DAY AS PARENTS OF AN AUTISTIC CHILD, AND I WAS CLUELESS AND SCARED.

What was I feeling on that fateful day? Honestly, I was generally numb to all of it. I did not know what it meant, so I did not know what to expect, what to fear, what to consider. It was enough to know my strong wife was falling apart in front of my eyes. The full effect of that day would not hit me for an extremely long time.

The pediatric neurologist that diagnosed Kyler tried to explain autism to us in simple terms. The autism developmental line is on a scale of 0 - 100. Zero is the most severe condition of autism with no retardation. 100 is still on the spectrum but fully able to function on one's own in the real world (the high end of Asperger's Syndrome). Zero would mean possibly needing to be institutionalized for the rest of one's life, and 100 would mean a person who was a bit weird, not fully comprehending the visual and non-spoken cues of social skills a normal person can decipher but able to be a self-sufficient adult with little or no assistance from others. So here is the bomb the doctor drops on us, our son is somewhere between a 5 and 10 on this imaginary 0-100 scale.

I digress. "No retardation" is a critical key here. We were blessed that no retardation was present at the age of 2 1/2, for that changes everything! Only a small percent of children diagnosed with severe autism do NOT have a form of retardation. We were blessed. I look at parents and families with children who have these disabilities, and I am grateful for my sons' condition. I applaud those parents whose children have such disabilities for their devotion to their child or children. The love of these parents is unconditional and unwavering. They should be given a medal, a standing ovation for the sacrifice and patience they must endure for the rest of their lives. Everyday they wake up not knowing what the world will throw at them but willing, always willing, to face it with an attitude of "I'm gonna make this day the best it can be." And then they go out and do it.

CHAPTER NINE

The Beginning:
Applied Behavioral Analysis and Gating

"As a child he screamed for hours on end never stopping, never abating. You can't know what that's like unless you've lived through it, and you have not lived through it."

"Sometimes I just want to scream. He might look normal but he's not. How do I make you believe that he understands about 25% of what you're saying?"

We have always been blessed when it came to finding the right person at the right time for Kyler. By referral from Paula and Gayle, we were put in touch with a behavioral specialist by the name of Fernando. We were assured that he would help with Kyler's behavior problems. We had shown that we were open to learning and would follow instructions. That is an important thing, because many parents do not want to hear that they are parenting wrong. They do not want to follow someone else's idea about how to raise their special needs child. I was one of those people, very sure that the way we were raising our children was the right way. We were successfully raising Brenna, and she was doing just fine. In fact, she was as close to the ideal child as she could get. I knew my boy was a bit difficult but he was a boy, the second child, and he had a slow start due to his hearing issues. We did not need any help. With my wife urging me to listen to this Fernando guy, I felt as though I had no choice but at least to act like I was going along. Begrudgingly I agreed to an introduction and meeting one night after a long day at work.

After our first meeting with Fernando, my wife decided it was best to try another approach to our child raising theories and put our faith in the professionals. We would do whatever they told us to do in order to help our son and ultimately our family. To say I was completely on board with what was going on would be far from the truth. In fact I was a bit resentful as to this approach my wife was taking, but with her being the stay at home mom and the person who was going to have to jump through the hoops, I followed her lead. My job was to go to work and provide for the family, and I was going to let her handle the stuff at home.

We did not know at the time, but when we invited Fernando into our home and lives, we were in for a rude awakening! It turned out Kyler was not the one who was in need of major behavior modification training. It was Dana and I who would have to unlearn everything we thought we knew about parenting. This was a major blow to my parenting ego!! As I have mentioned before, we had all our parenting plans worked out. We had planned and prepared ourselves for this time of our lives prior to having children, and now we were being told in straight out terms that we had no clue!! I did not want to hear that and I was not going to listen. Again my wife came to the rescue and said she would do it. She knew me and she knew in the beginning I was not going to be any part of the change. So here is Fernando's assessment: we were one of the reasons Kyler's behavior was unacceptable to us and to everyone else who encountered him in public. Now this is not to say it is our fault that Kyler is autistic, but it would be more correct to say that some of his behavioral problems had been magnified by our parenting methods. My heart dropped! I couldn't believe what I had just been told.

Our relationship with Fernando would go on for many years. Dana would become an ardent student of Fernando's parenting methods. She kept meticulous notes of his directions and did her very best to apply his recommendations in our parenting of Kyler.

So how did I play a part in Kyler's early development? I must honestly say I did little. I did not understand the problem with my boy nor did I fully understand the long term ramifications of his condition. When at home I did as I was instructed by my wife regarding Kyler's weekly action plan. When I would come home from work I would inquire or be told by my wife what Fernando had outlined for the week's development plans. Yes, I missed almost all those early planning meetings under the pretense that I needed to work. Although I was at work, I surely could have made some of the meetings. I was disinterested in this process, not disinterested in my son's development but disinterested because I still did not really understand how far behind my son was in his natural development as a toddler and how far he was falling behind day by day and month by month. Fortunately my wife did understand and she pushed that ball up the hill all by herself. The only thing I did right in those early years was not to push against her. I let her do what she felt was best for our son. Over the course of those early years, my wife's excellent student habits kicked in. She would eventually fill up three 3-inch 3-ring binders with notes and action plans developed by Fernando for Kyler's development team.

Fernando's official designation at that time by the State of Arizona was a behavior therapist. Under this title, any service he provided to us was covered by the state's DDD program. What we did not know about Fernando was that he was much more than a behavior therapist. In fact, he was a vastly over-qualified behavior modification therapist with many years of experience in applied behavioral analysis. He was working on his doctoral thesis on the topic. It just so happened while he was completing his education he moonlighted for the state as a behavior therapist. As it would turn out, Fernando would be the greatest influence on both our lives and that of our oldest son Kyler than any other of the over 100 therapists or professionals who would cross our path. We were very lucky to have caught Kyler's condition early. With our team of interventionists, Fernando at the lead, we were able to begin an intense applied behavioral analysis (ABA) program which would change the course of Kyler's life. (Note: Once we transitioned into the ABA program we did have to pay for Fernando's services as he led the team, but all the other habilitation services were covered by the state.) ABA is a treatment program which uses general principles of behavioral therapy to build skills that children with autism lack, such as language, social, academic, self-help, play, and attention skills. It also tries to minimize the unusual behaviors of kids with autism. Many studies and theories about this type of intervention support the notion that early intervention is the key to success in habilitating autistic kids to some degree. The best results in autistic habilitation have been conclusively shown when intensive therapies begin before the child is 32 months old. As luck would have it we started with Paula and occupational therapy (OT) when Kyler was 24 months.

Fernando told us what he was going to have us do would not be easy. In fact, it would be difficult, but if we did as he suggested we would see progress in Kyler, both in his behavior and his development. It took me much longer to accept my son's problem than my wife. It took a man telling me. Keep in mind I was raised in a traditional Hispanic household and as the man of the home I was not much into anyone coming into my home and telling me what I was doing was wrong and that I was the one who needed to change. That was just another reason we were so lucky to have Fernando as our behavioralist. I guess I needed to have another Hispanic male tell me that I had to forget my background and learn a new way that would aid my son and help him reach his full potential. I had to be willing to release control and listen to other people. I had to ignore bad behavior and not acknowledge it. I could not react when Kyler was being noisy or misbehaving. Man, did that go against everything in my own background and upbringing.

On that first visit with Fernando he asked us what we wanted to accomplish, what were the things Kyler was doing that we would like to see corrected? That was easy. We wanted to know how to get Kyler to stop the incessant screaming, throwing things, knocking over the trash, constant tantrums, and mashing his foods with his hands.

Let's start with the screaming. Fernando simply said to ignore him until he stops screaming. Our response was,"He never stops. He can scream for hours." Fernando said, "Then let him scream for hours. You have trained him how to behave and now you have to un-train him. *He has trained you well.*" We were shocked at that suggestion, and said we would give it a try. Fernando immediately said, "If you're simply going to give it a *try*, you will fail and my methods will not work." He told us curtly if we were not going to follow his directions to a "T" he was not going to work with us because we would fail. We now had three children: a 4, 3, and 8 month old. My wife was so exhausted with Kyler's behavior that she was willing to do anything to start moving in a new direction. From that day forward she dutifully did as we were told. How did it work out? We did not just give it a try; we did it. We had to commit 100 percent. Kyler would scream and we would ignore him. He would move to get in our face and scream and we would look right through him, slowly moving to look in another direction or continue our conversation. At no time were we to make eye contact. Once there was a break in the screaming (and in the beginning maybe he was just getting his breath) we would turn to him and nicely ask him what he needed. At that point we were ready to do anything he wanted.

It was an extremely difficult test run of Fernando's ideas, but if we were going to start getting better behavior out of Kyler we needed to try something different. However, it got much worse before it got better. Dana had to get ear plugs for when she was driving the car. She had over an hour commute multiple times a week to different therapists, and Kyler would scream and kick the seat the entire way.

In those early stages we had to demonstrate absolute, blind faith in the directions that were given to us by Fernando, and he promised us things would get much worse before they got better. That proved to be an understatement. No amount of warning could have prepare us for the onslaught of frustration and disruption that was going to envelop our home. We were about to turn Kyler's world upside down as we tried to force him to conform to the behavior we wanted and not to his accustomed behavior/existence. We later learned that not all families can do that, not because they don't want what is best for their child, but because it takes a large toll on all members of the family and their nerves over a fairly long period of time. It is not an easy path.

Our exceptional 4-year old daughter Brenna also had to be taught not to give in to Kyler. She was a great little helper and caught on quickly. But as I look back, I cannot believe what an amazing miracle she was in her ability to ignore Kyler. She was already way too mature for her age. As we continued to work on this project we were thrilled when there was a break in the screaming. We could only help Kyler when the screaming stopped. After a few weeks we extended the time of required silence between screaming and turning to help Kyler. When he would stop we would say things like "Good not screaming Kyler. What can I get you?" or "Kyler, how may I help you?" He did not understand the words we were using, but he did understand the tone of voice we were using. How long did this experiment last? Well... many agonizing months. Think of fingers scratching on the chalk board and how that would start to frazzle your nerves. Our nerves were more than frazzled. They were shredded. Eventually he stopped screaming and would come to get us, take us by the hand and lead us to what he wanted. After the years of screaming, we felt as though this was the greatest miracle ever. We were also trying to teach him simple sign language. Dana made cards with pictures on them (Pec cards) that he could point to, so he could let us know what he wanted or needed.

As with all learning this was a building block process, and to stop the screaming was the first of those blocks to be laid. Communication would come next using sign language and picture cards. Many months had passed but real communication had begun and we were ecstatic.

Throwing everything was also on our first Fernando list. How to get him to stop? What we learned was that Kyler threw things because he did not know how to play with them. "WHAT?" was my reaction. How could he not know how to play? That's ridiculous. Kids are innately able to play. I clearly still did not understand what we were dealing with. We had been told this by the first speech therapist, Nina, but I had not believed or truly understood what she was trying to convey. We were not the kind of parents who had lots of toys around for the kids to play with. Our incorrect assumption was that kids could use their imagination to play and did not need lots and lots of toys that in all honesty we thought just made a mess. But what if you do not have an imagination? Then what? Well Kyler did not have much going on up in that head of his. At 30-34 months his age appropriate level, as measured by his primary care physician, was at 6-9 months. So he screamed and threw things. Both of which he was very good at. So how do you teach a 3-year old child, at a 6-9 month old learning level, how to play? Much like the screaming, it was done slowly and painfully, one skill at a time. Gating and lots of positive reinforcement became our mantra.

What is gating? The Merriam-Webster official definition would be, "*An action, process, or mechanism by which the passage of something is controlled.*" Gating for the purposes of our situation simply put was our way to encourage Kyler to do things the way we wanted him to do by denying him things he wanted until his behavior was in line with what we wanted. It was a reward system set up to make it worth his while to cooperate with any activity. We all use gating as parents but we do not do it for each and every action. If a child wants a cell phone then get good grades and we will get you one, or if you're good at church we will get you an ice cream later. With normal children we often use gating but we are hardly ever consistently doing it for all of the actions of a child. With Kyler this was different. Every action and desired progression on his part had to be gated. Finding the things that motivated him was difficult in the beginning. He had the mind of a 6-9 month old, and what does a 6-9 month old want? Food, water, no gas in the stomach, a clean bottom, a little visual stimulation, and movement. That was Kyler at 32 months old.

So, how did we get Kyler to start playing with toys? It started with the easy wooden puzzles that have pictures with little knobs on them. Of course we did not have any so we went out and bought some. We would help him put them in place and make a big production each time one went in. There were many times in the beginning when it was us playing with the puzzles and Kyler doing some heavy movement in the room, like jumping off stuff or falling down or any other physically demanding activity. As jumping on the furniture like a trampoline was usually not allowed, it drove us crazy to have to ignore that behavior and act like we were having the time of our lives playing with those simple puzzles. We would high five and make a big deal about our getting the puzzle right. On the rare occasions I was home, I would sit with my wife doing those things, thinking that it was pure nonsense. How could our playing without him help him learn to start playing with puzzles? But, after the screaming started to abate, (I had agreed to follow Fernando to the letter) I played along. I was not sure that I was doing the right thing, but Kyler's screaming was getting much better so maybe this might work too. As we were playing, Kyler would get no positive or negative reinforcement for his behavior unless he was involved in the puzzle. He would come around to play with us, and we would first make a big deal about his coming to join us. Then if he got a piece in, often with our help, we would clap and be excited. After many weeks Kyler started to want to do the puzzles. However, here is the rub. Kyler had to be taught how to insert each and every piece of the puzzle as though each piece was an entirly different puzzle unto itself. He had to be taught how to play with each piece of every toy or game. He could not learn by watching us or other kids play with certain toys then mimic them. He could not transfer knowledge from one activity to another. We had to take the time to teach him how to play with each toy. This teaching would take hours or even days with each toy.

This is where our habilitation worker, Shawn, came into play. She was our miracle, our angel. She came to our home 30-40 hours a week, 50 weeks a year, to work on our (ABA) Applied Behavioral Analysis Plan set up by our team of professionals with Fernando as the lead. In the beginning we would video and have bi-monthly meetings and set up an action plan that had her working on specific tasks with Kyler. Fernando would watch the video and give feedback on what was done right, what was done wrong, and what new stuff needed to be taught. Much of the training was like Pavlov's dog. We would reward Kyler for acceptable behavior and ignore everything else. The trick was finding what he wanted. What was his "gate"? Graham crackers, M&M's, swimming, cookies, jumping on the frog swing, all became wonderful rewards for appropriate actions. Kyler started to learn step-by-step, action-by-action what we wanted him to do. Due to his strictly rote behavior learning, all actions had to be taught, retaught, and then re-reinforced until it became a part of his behavior.

Shawn was so patient and willing to learn. She listened to everything Fernando told her and implemented it to the best of her ability. Every day she would come and work diligently on the current action plan of the week. Every activity was focused on that plan. There would be other trainers later in Kyler's life, Galite, Sara, Isabel, Kathy, and John, but Shawn had the most impact on Kyler. Those trainers would be in our home for the next eight years. After third grade, Kyler's habilitation time went down to 15-20 hours a week.

Our last item on that first list we wanted Fernando to fix was the weird things Kyler did at meal time. Remember he threw everything and also mutilated his food. We learned he was craving sensory input. He also "chipmunked" his food. We never found out why he did that but we learned to clean out his mouth after meal time. We were taught two things. One, if food is available kids will not starve themselves, but just barely. Two, odds are Kyler was going to eat only a selective diet and we had to find out what that was. I was not okay with the notion that we needed to find out what he wanted. I was raised that you eat what was put in front of you or you don't eat. Now I was being told to cater to my 3-year old son? That was not how I was raised nor what I believed at my core, but other experiments were working, so how could I buck the system on these issues? Over the years a few of the things he will eat have changed, but we quickly learned his picky diet had a lot to do with the texture of the food and less to do with the taste. He would even eat some bland foods as long as the texture was soft. This still holds true today 15 years later. For example, he likes pancakes but he will eat them only after they have been left to sit under a large bowl and allowed to go soft, especially on the edges, otherwise he will eat only the middle and leave the outsides. Of course the pancakes and syrup have to be a particular brand. Not just any brand can be used. He knows the difference.

Another question for Fernando was, "How do we get him to stop throwing his food?" The answer: Give him only one portion at a time and if he threw it he would get no more. No scolding, no force feeding, no begging, no reinforcement at all with regard to his behavior. He would eat when he was hungry enough to eat.

Of course, change is never easy, so that new feeding tactic came with a major downside: we experienced a new round of incessant screaming. That had to be dealt with in the prescribed way, and in the end it did work. As for the mutilation of food, once we learned about his sensory needs we started providing him ways to get that input. Some of those included: playing in sand, buckets of pinto beans, shaving cream, small pebble rocks, mud, workout balls, swings, and this list went on. Of course those things could be thrown, so as you can guess, there was more removal of the things he wanted and more screaming. We stayed consistent to what we were being told to do and consistent in how we handled his behavior and after a couple of months things started to get better. I did not say things were better. His behavior slowly started to change and to improve. We worked on speech to start communicating, but really it was sign language and picture cards (pec cards) that were to be his first signs of communication.

CHAPTER TEN

A Dad's Maturation

"I live in constant fear. Will they make good decisions when crossing the road and getting on a bus or walking down the street or riding a bike? I know these are the same questions regular parents ask themselves, but it's not to be a question they have to ask themselves their entire lives as I will."

I think about a boy I knew in school who was, as they said back then, "slow." He never did anything bad to others, minded his own business, went to class, and stayed out of our way. Special classes were provided for these kids, "resource classes." Were we nice to him? No, not really. Did we tease him sometimes? Yes, I regret to say we did. We never hurt him physically but I shudder to think what we may have done to him emotionally. Now that was possibly going to be the life of my boy, my son, my pride. How was/am I going to save him from that pain, from the humiliation and shame he may have to endure at the hands of others? How was I going to deal with other people's insults and abuse of my son? Just the thought of those possible actions of others made me angry, made me feel pain, left me feeling shame for how I had treated that boy in junior high. Though never the ring leader, I was a participant and this brought me to a painful inner reflection that I cannot describe.

So what about my son? What was I going to do? How was I going to do it? The realization of how my hopes and dreams had to change for my son took place in stages. Initially, I did not really know what the diagnosis of severe autism meant. This would come only with time and with a realization of what Kyler's successes were in comparison to those of a "normal" child. This slow realization of his development delay also turned out to be a blessing. We have never settled for good enough with Kyler. Even though we came to accept that his condition would be set by some unknown boundary, we did not know what that boundary was, so our expectations were to push for as much progress in development as possible and the boundary of his ability to learn and get better would make itself known when we got there. I believe that is why he has done so well, relatively speaking. We never stopped expecting more from him, his trainers, his teachers, and more importantly from ourselves.

We have always realized how fortunate we were in putting together such a dedicated group of team leaders, teachers, and trainers for Kyler. Not many families can say that, and as you will later see we were not as lucky the second time with Koleden, but for Kyler we were.

Maybe more important than changing Kyler and helping him to reach his full potential, I was the one who was going to be in for the most internal change. I had to accept that I was the father of a son who would be and is different. I was not going to enjoy some of the father milestones of pride. I was not going to have an All-Star athlete son. I was not going to be the father of a son who achieved greatness in the classroom. My son was not going to be the most popular kid in school. My son was not going to be a leader of boys and men. I was not going to have the career I had always envisioned for myself. I was not going to be able to travel as my wife and I always dreamed about. I would have to settle for something personally and professionally below what I had set as my own personal goal. One may ask why I was settling for mediocrity with my personal goals. I would say I was not settling; I was just reformulating. I strongly felt my son's development took priority, and I was going to do everything I could to make that happen.

Having a special needs child comes with a certain amount of internal introspection. I would often spend hours considering my situation and how I might have been responsible for Kyler's condition. As earlier mentioned, I have been fairly successful in sports, school, business, life, and now I fathered a son who would be none of these. What kind of failure was I? Did I give him a bad gene? What did I do that may have caused him to have this condition? Should I have been better prepared as a father to deal with his issues? Could we have caught his condition earlier and been farther along in the development process? Why was this happening to me and my family? What did I do to cause all of this? I think you see where this is going. My thoughts were about me, about how all this was going to affect me and my dreams. I was being selfish, but how can you not feel all these things? Every time a father holds his new baby boy in his hands, these are the types of things he ponders concerning the future of his son. It is only natural to feel this way. But this was not to be for me and my son. Kyler's path would be markedly different from the one I had envisioned. That does not mean it is a future we do not make every effort to improve upon and enhance by way of understanding what we can do to assist him every step of the way. We decided we had to go in a new direction in life. We had to put aside some of our personal career and parenting hopes and dreams and allow some of that focus to go into our boy, my boy.

So the beginning was underway. Fernando had started us on a path of rehabilitation, not just for Kyler but also for us, for me. I slowly came to understand we had to change our parenting style and our expectations for the future.

CHAPTER ELEVEN

WHERE IS KYLER?

*"When he hears people screaming, he internalizes and feels
as though they are stabbing him with daggers, even if it's
positive screaming."*

Most autistic children are escape artists. They are able to find ways
to get out of almost anything. They have no need for anyone, so they
wander off without the fear of being away from a parent. This being
said, "Where is Kyler?" became as common a phrase as it is to take
a breath. He could put some distance between us in a heartbeat.
We could not go anywhere without always having one eye on Kyler.
Whether at the pool, ballgame, family party, or even at home, the
constant question at least 10 times an hour was "Where is Kyler?" We
even put security locks high up on every door of our house and yard
to make sure he could not escape. Even with all those precautions
he still found ways to escape. He was an expert. From the time he
could walk until about the age of 8, Kyler demonstrated no fear of
anything. Getting lost was not something he considered. Getting
hurt was the farthest thing from his mind. I guess the truth is there
was not a lot going on in his mind other than the most basic needs of
the body: food, water, some sleep (not much), and I guess what was
on the TV. Everything else had no place or need in his world. At one
point we even looked into getting a tracking device inserted under
the skin so that when he escaped us, we would be able to find him.

I suppose all parents go through these worries and concerns at
periods of their children's lives, but it truly is different with a special

needs child. There is no way to explain why or how it is. When you go to a ball field of any kind, the first thing you make a note of is where are the gates or possible exits? Do you go to people's homes and sit where you can see the front door so that you have the escape route covered? It is not uncommon to see families at Disneyland with their small kids on a leash, but do you like walking around Disneyland with a leash on your 8-yr old and the leash being held by your 9-yr old daughter? Again this can be a bit embarrassing because people look at you and you know (in your own mind) that they are judging you and wondering what kind of parent are you? Do you go to church and have to hold your 8-yr old child in your lap because if you don't he will escape and go who knows where? Do you not go to movies, trips, family outings, families' homes, ballgames, restaurants, fairs, friends' homes, plays, etc. because it's not worth the embarrassment or trouble involved with the constant worry that goes along with any outing of any kind.

I have a good friend who has a daughter with Down Syndrome. She is sweet and loving but you can tell by looking at her face that she is different, a special gift from our Father in Heaven. One day she escaped the house. They live in a rural area where homes are on 10-40 acre lots. Their home has all the same safeguards we have to keep our young Kyler in. She escaped to a neighbor's house and went inside and started helping herself to some goodies in the refrigerator. The neighbors came home and found her safe and sound. In the meantime the alarm bells had been sounded and for 20-minutes my friends were going crazy looking for her. Then the phone rang and they were told she was at their neighbor's house 1/4 mile away, safe and sound.

Now if the same type of thing had happened to my 8-year old Kyler, people would look at us like "control your kid," because while he looks normal he acts different. It's hard to deal with all the judgement or perceived judgement of others around you. On another occasion there was a time when my wife was out with Kyler and he had a meltdown. She was taking him out of the store kicking and screaming with Brenna walking beside her when a woman told her what a horrible parent she must be and how she needed to learn how to parent and control her child. Dana left the store crying and did so all the way home. These pronounced judgements by others, although ignorant in their statement, still can be hurtful.

I could go on for pages about these types of events, and I know all parents experience some types of gut wrenching moments with some of their kids on occasions. But for us it was a constant dilemma that made us have to think very carefully before we considered going out anywhere. And worse, no matter how hard we tried, we could not get our extended families to understand what we were going through. It made me so mad sometimes that I wanted to lecture them, to make them understand, but it was no use. All they could see were two boys who *look* normal, so they should *be* normal. I know this is surprising considering the pervasiveness of autism in our society today, but there it is, not sugar coated, just a fact that many parents of autistic children must endure.

Our own famlies have also failed us in this area, not that they do not know the boys are autistic, but because so many of them have never invested the time to try and understand what this condition means. They have not had a book like this to give them an insight into the lives of an autistic family. This said we do have two family members out of over fifty whom have come to unconditionally accept the boys for who they are and just try to be their friend. The boys love them for this, for their basic level of friendship. The boys love being around these two and look forward to times when they can be with them. We wish we could say that about all our family members.

The following are some examples of actual situations that have happened with our boys. Many people will read these stories and think to themselves, "These are common occurances with all children," and this is true. But not many parents investigate/research the possibility of injecting a tracking device in their child, or decide it is better to avoid going out because they are so worried they will lose their child in a split second of distraction. And as the child gets older they get faster and can put more distance between you and them in a heartbeat. Sometimes it's just easier to stay home.

Losing Kyler at a birthday party
As usual we had one eye on Kyler as we spent time with our family at my niece's birthday party. Kyler was 2 1/2-years old. We were at a very large apartment complex that had a large grassy park and swimming pool in the middle of the complex next to a major roadway. As usual I made a quick assessment of the area and escape routes. Dana and I developed a sort of non-spoken communication system inquiring constantly "Where's Kyler? Do you see him?" It just became the way we did things when we were out.

At one point in the party it became time to hit the Piñata. This is a common Hispanic tradition. A piñata is often a paper mâché cartoon character that is filled with candy and toys. It is hoisted in the air by a rope, usually, and then the children by age and size get to hit it with a stick. Starting with the youngest and smallest, the child is blindfolded and turned in 3 circles. They are then presented to the piñata by having the stick tapped against it by a helper. They are given three chances to strike it and send all the candy flying. Most children can't wait for this to start, and it is always a favorite event for the parents to watch. So in preparation for the piñata, the men were getting things put together. We had no rope and used a set of battery cables. (Hey, we're Mexicans. We improvise.) My brother climbed high up a tree to control the piñata. This took about 7-10 minutes to get organized. As we finished getting ready, Dana and I made eye contact and asked each other "Where's Kyler?" We quickly scanned the kids, nothing. We scanned the general area, nothing. We started asking everyone if they had seen Kyler. The family was so engrossed in the game that they did not notice our panic and really offered no help, because they could not imagine any child not just being thrilled with the pinata. Then Dana spotted him. He was 150-yards away heading into the parking lot. Dana was already 50-yards ahead of me and sprinting, so I grabbed the video camera and got her catching up with him.

My father asked me what was wrong with my kid that he just went off like that. He insisted that well-trained and behaved children do not do that. And why didn't he like to hit the piñata? Those kinds of comments can be frustrating and painful. You learn to disregard them when they come from strangers or the looks you get from strangers, but when your family does it, it just hurts. They are judging your parenting skills when they have no idea how much work it is to raise an autistic child who has zero comprehension of what is going on around him. In the case of this party he wanted nothing to do with anyone there. This is not because he does not like them but because he just has no connection to them. He exists in his own world, and no one else is there with him.

So how did I deal with this? Just like a good obedient Hispanic son should; I bit my tongue and sheepishly mumbled something about how Kyler just likes to be by himself. I felt that if I tried to explain to my dad in a few words what was happening to his grandson it would have been a waste of my breath. Not to mention I really had only a small grasp of Kyler's condition at that time. Over the years I have tried to educate my father and all my extended family for that matter, with varying amounts of success, but to say any of them are quazi-experts or well informed about the condition would not be accurate.

The time I lost Kyler in the mountain
Losing Kyler is not only a fear but also a reality that due to dumb luck did not end too tragically. When Kyler was 3 1/2, our church had an overnight outing for fathers and sons at a nearby mountain campsite. I had camped many times as a youth in the area and felt I could keep a pretty good eye on him. Dana was concerned because she knew how quickly Kyler could disappear. She warned me not to take my eyes off of him. The night went well as I kept him close and we got a good night's sleep in the back of our locked SUV. In the morning it was time to eat. The older men in the group were making pancakes, Kyler's favorite breakfast. I waited patiently with Kyler for our turn of pancakes to come up. I left Kyler sitting at a table 20 feet away and went and got our food. I went to the butter and syrup station to get everything ready and turned back to the table to eat with Kyler. Once I turned, my worst fear was realized, "Kyler was gone."

At this point in his life Kyler did not respond to his name, but I yelled out for him anyway. He was basically non-verbal with a few sign language gestures. I looked frantically around the open area but no Kyler. There were 15-20 people in the area as some of the other men and boys had gone off to do some hiking and caving. So a quick scan around clearly showed there was no Kyler anywhere. I started to panic and made a quick run around the perimeter of the camping area, a space about 40-yards wide and 60-yards long. Still no sign of him and 5-7 minutes had passed since I last saw him. I knew this could get bad. As he had no fear of anything and no realization of danger, I was worried he could go a great distance very quickly. I had seen this before and I was truly becoming scared. I knew if I lost him my wife would be crazy angry. I was embarrassed to ask some of the men around me to help me search for him. People have never understood Kyler's disability, partly because he just looks so normal. Most of them think all boys have his issues, so I was worried what these men would say. Perhaps they might think I was crying wolf. So, I continued to keep looking by myself, getting more and more physically ill with every passing minute. Twenty minutes passed and I had looked everywhere more than once: up the dry creek 75-yards and down the dry creek 75-yards. I had asked a few people if they had seen him but not many of them really knew who he was. I was at my wits end, so I said a short prayer and decided it was time to get some help. I was very embarrassed to ask for help but if too much more time passed, who knows how far he could get from his starting point. I was heading back to the center of activity to get a search party started when I spotted him just wandering around near the end of the clearing. I ran to him and picked him up and held him tight and hugged him. I asked him where he had been, but he did not understand the question or that I was worried about him. He was just there in body. He had no idea what had just happened. I got home and fessed up to my wife about the incident. She admitted she would have been angry with me for losing him, but she also understood how it had all happened so quickly.

Kyler going down a river:
When Kyler was 4, my family had a reunion on the banks of the Gila River. It was a one day event and there were about 60 people there. My wife was extremely concerned because we had four kids ages 5 and under. Our youngest was an infant and able to be in the playpen, but that left our two boys, 20-months and 4-years, and our oldest at age 5. This is a very dangerous, fast moving river because there is a lot of undertow and a lot of debris in the water. I really wanted to float down it with my 7 siblings and numerous cousins, but my wife refused to let me. Her excuse was that she could not watch all four kids by herself around such a river. Her dad had been an Adventure P.E. teacher and she had been down this river many times and knew the dangers of the river. She needed me to help her watch the kids. Of course, I was not really happy with her, but I agreed.

I had not accepted Kyler's condition yet, so my attitude was one of, "You can take care of all the kids; I really want to go down the river." As you can guess it was not the most harmonious of trips for my family. Anyway, once my siblings came down the river, everyone was laughing and having fun. They were not watching their tubes. Dana had her hands full trying to keep her eye on Koleden, Brenna, and Kyler. I was socializing with my family since I didn't get to go down the river with them. I left most of the parenting of the kids up to my wife unless she asked for help. That was not something I am proud of; it was just easier for me to escape that way. Suddenly she cried out to me that she had lost sight of Kyler. Immediately I began searching. I yelled to my family to search. Luckily my brother Ani saw Kyler on a tube about 30 yards down river and he took off running. We all started screaming for other people to stop that little boy. All the people on the banks of the river were jumping in trying to get to him. Dana and I kept screaming for him not to let go. It was one of the most scary moments of my life. My brother Ani was the one to catch him and drag him to shore. I hated to admit it, but my wife had been right!

Kyler almost jumps off Havasu Falls

When Kyler was 5-years old we decided to take him and Brenna on a trip to the Grand Canyon with family. I had reservations about this, keeping in mind Kyler did not speak much and understood very little that was said to him. He feared nothing, but my fear was that he might go to the edge of the abyss and jump in just to see what it felt like. "No fear" was not just a saying for Kyler but a state of existence. We made the 12-mile hike to Havasupi Falls on the first day, and Kyler did surprisingly well. When we finally got to the falls, all of us in the party were ready to soak our tired feet in the cool aqua blue water. I had sprained my ankle on the trip down the canyon so when I got to the water I couldn't wait to take my shoe off and soak my foot. For one fleeting moment I took my eye off Kyler. A couple of minutes passed and my internal clock said it was time to ask that constant question, "Where's Kyler?" I was watching the lagoon around the base of the waterfalls the entire time, so I knew he was not there. I first glanced around the open area down the small river and still no Kyler. From experience I knew it was time to sound the alarm. My wife had the same internal clock and had been scanning the area, first the pool then the open area, and quickly we realized Kyler was nowhere to be found. From previous experience we knew our search must expand fast. We quickly told everyone in the group to start looking for Kyler. My brother-in-law Tom spotted him ascending the path half way back up the mountain where the falls come over the cliff. That was a 121-foot drop. We all called after Kyler and he stopped and turned, pointing up to the top of the cliff, and just kept moving up the hill. My other brother-in-law, Lincoln, was closer so he started running up the hill to catch Kyler. We managed to slow Kyler down by calling his name and having him look back at us. Lincoln ran up the hill and finally caught up with Kyler just as he got to the edge of the river at the top of the cliff. Lincoln grabbed him and brought him back down. When Kyler was finally delivered to Dana, she asked him where he was going. His response was typical Kyler, only one word: "JUMP" while he pointed to the top of the falls. Our hearts about dropped.

"No fear" is not just a saying for some autistic kids. They truly cannot comprehend that anything can hurt them. They are scared of nothing because in their world nothing means anything to them.

CHAPTER TWELVE
REACHING FOR THE SKY

"His social skills are very limited. If he's in a new situation he doesn't know how to act appropriately."

"He is intelligent in that he can be taught any thing; it just takes time to teach and a lot of repetition. Teaching the same topic in different ways can be difficult for the teacher, but he can be taught."

From the beginning when people would tell us how well Kyler was doing, we did not want to hear it. It was not that we were not pleased with his progress, we were excited about every newly achieved milestone, but often these comments would come from people who were looking through what we felt were rose colored glasses. They were usually emphasizing what he was doing right and not what we could be working on or how he could improve. When it came to dealing with the school system working with Kyler, we often found people were afraid to upset us with negatives or discuss areas of concerns. This was especially true when dealing with teachers. We always set our bar of expectations for Kyler just out of reach so that we were always shooting for the ever elusive achievements that would propel Kyler toward being somewhere near "normal." We also set the bar high for everyone who was working with him. We expected more; we demanded progress; we forced teachers to do things that Fernando advocated. We were generally a major pain in the neck with all the accommodations that we expected from those who were working with Kyler to help in his development. We learned that we had to become his advocate. Good was not going to be good enough for my Kyler. To achieve this, he would have to be pushed and the people pushing him had to be pushed.

Just because Kyler had been labeled within the autistic spectrum did not mean we did not have expectations for our son. We were not going to allow him to sit in a corner day after day rocking himself, playing/shaking his hands in front of his face, or hitting himself. That was not acceptable, so what were our expectations? After much thought and research about autism we decided to aim high. If we fell short it would still be a great improvement over where he began. We wanted him to be the best that he could be, perhaps even "normal." In retrospect, I now know that was not going to be possible, but I do not regret this being the goal because this attitude propelled us forward and upward.

What were our expectations or goals for Kyler? Dana and I spent countless hours considering that over the period of several years. We tried to read books and periodicals that would give us a clue as to what we could expect. We watched many TV specials that were airing because of the pandemic-like rise in the number of autistic children per 1,000 that were being diagnosed. Today autistic statistics are not measured in how many per 1,000 but how many per less than 100 and dropping. One thing we could not find was what we could expect or hope Kyler's outcome to be. What was the end-game? We came up with our own goals/expectations/dreams. There were always many little subgoals for every main goal. Of course we would meet with our team and set mini-weekly, monthly, and yearly goals that we would strive to meet.

Our first main long term goal was to get Kyler to participate in a mainstream classroom. Our next main goal was to help him develop to the point that if anyone were to encounter him on the street, in a classroom, or on a playground, after observing him for some time, that person would say, "Hey, there is something that's just not quite right with that kid," even though he would not be able to put his finger on it. These were our goals/expectations/dreams and we made sure everyone around us knew it. Settling for anything less would be to let Kyler fail and that was not an option.

Today I would say we have generally succeded in our main goals. Although Kyler's cognitive and interpersonal skills are extremely delayed, his ability to mimic and model those around him are exceptional. He is not generally disruptive or a nuisance and is very good at just acting and blending in. Sometimes I wonder if we did the right thing because he can be so "normal" looking that people discriminate against him. For example, when he does not always follow directions given to him, people just don't understand he doesn't get it. They think he is being lazy or disrespectful. They think he is doing it on purpose. He would never tell them that he does not understand.

CHAPTER THIRTEEN
What Do Other People Think?

*"He's a great kid and doesn't cause any trouble.
That doesn't mean he is normal."*

*"Sometimes I wish he had a look which told you
immediately there was something not right. At least then I
wouldn't have to always be trying to explain."*

Unfortunately, like so many parents, I used to put a lot of stock in
what other people thought. As I have stated before, our first child
Brenna was as near a perfect little angel as could be. I could take her
anywhere and she would just make any parent proud at how well she
behaved. In the grocery store she would flirt with the people in line,
talking to anyone, and being just so engaging. Kyler was another
story. When we would take him out anywhere we were always
hyper-aware of his tantrums and his "acting out." In the early years I
felt he was being belligerent and disobedient. We might be walking
down an aisle and he would throw things out of the basket or start
screaming for no reason. As I have mentioned before, this was no
small scream but a very loud high pitched sound that literally made
your ears hurt. And of course it made everyone turn and watch. I
knew just what they were thinking, "Can't they control their kid?" or
"Shut him up would you?" or "What bad parents they must be," or "I
know how I would handle that kid if he were mine," or "Don't bother
us with your kid if you can't control him," or "Take him outside until
you get him under control." The stares, the looks, the shaking of
heads, the whispers, oh it was so embarrassing and humiliating

that I just did not want to take him anywhere. My pride and joy, my son, was not living up to the high standards/expectations I had envisioned. I felt the pain and frustration at my core, deep down, where no one wants to look, especially as a new father of a son. After we had been to the OT and knew there would be struggles, all those opinions were made worse. I wanted to yell and scream at all those people to cut me and my son some slack. He was not normal and we were both struggling with how to deal with it.

On yet another occasion a woman approached my wife and told her how bad a parent she was and that she shouldn't have children if she couldn't control her son. It happened to be a checkup day with Kyler's doctor. My wife told the doctor of the event and the doctor actually got angry. She commented that the woman had no idea what we were facing and how much we were doing to help Kyler. How dare she make judgements about us? I wish that were true, but sadly, human nature is to judge first and ask questions later.

Diaper boy:
When Kyler was 3-years old we went to our community pool. He was still not potty trained so we had him in swimmies. This would protect everyone else in the pool in case of an accident. At the pool he loved to splash in the water and jump into my waiting arms. We learned that the heavy pressure of his body hitting the water was very soothing for him, so we made every effort to take him to the pool as often as possible. On one particular day he tried to play with some other kids. They spotted the diaper and started making fun of him. They ran away from him and called him "diaper boy." To Kyler this was a great game, he chased and they ran. Kyler chased and laughed and laughed. The other kids ran from the boy with a diaper, just being kids, mean spirited, but just kids all the same. We watched in pain as if looking to the future of what his life could and probably would be like, ridiculed for his difference, for his inability to understand what was going on around him. We watched, not

interfering, knowing this would be something he would someday have to endure on his own without us there to protect him, but for now all was well. Kyler had no clue he was being made fun of, that no one wanted to play with him or be near him. His comprehension was barely a few words, and he had no understanding of what was happening, but we did and it hurt to watch. It was very painful. His future was going to be hard and full of uphill battles, and we knew it. These types of events lead to more sleepless nights and questioning of ourselves. Were we doing the right things for Kyler? Were we doing enough to help him?

CHAPTER FOURTEEN
THE GREAT AMERICAN PASTIME

"I don't know how many different ways to say it, but he cannot cross information from one situation to another. Every situation in his life is new and has to be figured out and categorized in his brain."

"He's a good-looking kid with some athletic ability. This confuses people because they just don't understand that all the synapses are not firing in his brain."

This leads me to his/our foray into Little League baseball. As I have mentioned before, it has taken me many years to come to an understanding of what Kyler's thresholds of success would be. I was lucky enough to be able to coach Kyler for most of his Little League career. When Kyler was 5-years old I knew he was ahead of his peers in gross motor skills and eye-hand coordination after just the first practice. What I was still in denial about was my understanding of how his ability to comprehend and follow directions would affect his head start in natural athletic ability. He had been going to school since the age of three but had not started kindergarten yet, so I was not yet aware of his lack of general comprehension compared with other kids his age.

Tee ball can be a very cute activity with kids hitting the ball and running to the bases. On rare occasions an exceptional player will field the ball and make a play at first. Even more rare is the child who has a grasp of the game and makes plays all over the field, catching fly balls, fielding balls, tagging out runners, and getting force plays at the appropriate bases. Well I taught Kyler to do just a few things and after a lot of work he was able to do some simple tasks pretty well. One was to hit the ball, then run to just one base, then checking with the coach to see if he should run to the next base. Because he was the best hitter on the team he often hit last and would be told to run, run, run. This he did fairly well and I knew he was on his way to being "normal." Okay, I was the one who felt this way. But he could hit and run so well, better than 90% of the kids out there. I kept telling myself that he was going to be fine.

I was brought back to my senses when Kyler was in the field. Over time I came to realize that Kyler could not understand directions that were given to the team in general. If he was told to do something in a group setting, he flat out could not comprehend _anything_ that was being said. So with his great arm, I taught him how to play the pitcher position and second base. His directions were clear and always the same: catch the ball and throw it to first. I was quite successful with this approach, but when situations required a different play, he could not grasp what we wanted. I learned that we as coaches could not change his directions in the middle of a game. We now know that his learning is 100% rote only. Everything he learns is by rote repetition, and if we do not spend a significant amount of time on a specific action, he cannot learn it. So teaching him over and over always to catch the ball and throw it to first was great, and over time he did learn this. He was not developing an understanding of the game of baseball; he was only learning a rote reaction to an event. I also learned through this that if I changed the directions to his predetermined rote behavior, I was in essence erasing the action he had learned up to that point. So I learned to keep it simple and give him one task to do over and over again so that he could be successful. I got to be the proud dad of the kid out there hitting the ball and making plays. I guess we once again see that ever present big elephant in the room—my ego, my dreams, my inability to accept my son's disability.

Tee-ball led to coach's pitch. I spent a lot of time teaching Kyler to hit whiffle balls in the backyard, and because of this, he continued to be one of the best players on his team. I continued to teach him how to play second base, but his comprehension of the game did not improve much. I started to teach him to play the catcher position since too many decisions had to be made at second base. What I did learn from this time is that with 50 times more repetition than what it took a regular kid, Kyler could start to understand what he should do. It still had to be kept simple. For example, he struggled to understand why in some cases he had to tag the runner when he was running to the base, and on other occasions all he had to do was touch the base when it was a force out situation. After 7 years of playing baseball he never really understood that concept while in the flow of a game. This being said, he was playing coach's pitch and the level of understanding by most of the kids playing on his team, did not outweigh his physical ability level, and he was still able to compete successfully. At this point I kept saying to myself that my son was going to be fine. My dreams for him would come true. He would continue to develop and turn out to be a really good baseball player.

Coach's pitch leads to the minor leagues. This is the level below the normal Little League play. Over time I had taught Kyler how to play catcher and to pitch. He threw pretty hard for a kid his age and with lots of practice I taught him how to pitch off the mound with a wind up. He even learned how to throw a knuckle ball, which was more like a change that did not spin. I taught him the knuckler because he liked what it looked like when I threw them at him while just playing catch. So for the next three years he played minor Little League. My son was going to be fine. My dream for him would come true, because he continued to excel at my favorite game, BASEBALL.

His hitting took a big blow in his second year of minor Little League. A wild pitch hit him in the back of the neck just below the helmet. Bad luck would have it that the kid who threw this pitch was the hardest throwing kid in the league. Kyler was never again the same at the plate after that happened. He could hit well if the opposing pitcher did not throw hard, but once he was facing a better pitcher with more velocity, he was just too afraid to stay in there and swing. His pitching on the other hand became his strong suit. As he got older he could throw harder and with good accuracy. As an 11-year old he was playing with kids 1-2 years younger and he was the dominant pitcher on our team. He led the team to a second place finish in a three league playoff. Wow, was I proud of what my son was accomplishing in sports! This was not supposed to happen but it did, and I was excited for him and for me. My son was going to be fine. My dream for him was going to come true.

Kyler turned 12 and that meant it was time to move up to Little League, the Majors. I had him placed on a team with a good coach who I asked to keep an eye on him. I told the coach that I was realistic about Kyler's playing level, but I felt he could be a good 9th or 10th man who might be able to provide him the odd inning of pitching if he was in a jam with available innings some weeks. This proved to be an accurate assessment. Kyler was subbed in and out playing the minimum required innings and minimum at bats. He did get to pitch a few times and though he was not dominate he did get some strikeouts and ate up the odd innings.

Kyler's organized baseball career came to a tragic end one evening at practice. He was involved in infield practice, playing 3rd base. The drill had Kyler rotating out while the other 3rd baseman was taking his turn. At the end of the drill the catcher was to throw the ball back to the attending third baseman. The catcher made a wild throw. Kyler was standing well behind third base watching the outfield taking fly balls when the errant ball struck Kyler in the back of the head. As fate would have it, it was the same hard throwing young man that had hit Kyler in the back of the neck a few years earlier. Of course it was an accident, and had Kyler been paying attention it would not have happened, but it did. This turned out to be quite a traumatic event in Kyler's life. The ball had hit him with such force that it cracked his skull and caused bleeding and bruising on the brain. It was so serious that Kyler spent several days in intensive care under observation at the Children's Hospital in a major city 100 miles away. His baseball career was now over. He was too afraid to continue. I must admit there was a part of me that wanted/held out a small hope that maybe, just maybe, I could get him to the point where he could pitch in high school. It was a small pipe dream, but it was a dream I had all the way back to the day he was born. Now it was surely gone. My son was *not* going to be okay. My baseball dreams for him were *not* going to come true.

It was about the time of Kyler's serious head injury that one of my best friends had an epiphany concerning our different lives. Just at that time my second son, Koleden, was diagnosed with late onset autism. His realization brought it all into focus for him and had a profound effect on me, because it came from an outsider looking in. To understand the incident, you need to know that this friend has three sons, all of whom were above average 3-sport high school athletes, really good students, and great young men. I attended many of their games and witnessed many of their greatest athletic accomplishments. They are now grown men with families of their own, but they still refer to me as their "Uncle."

We were having lunch one day discussing his boys and the young grandchildren he now had, when the topic turned to my boys and their cloudy futures or prospects. He said to me in more of a statement than a question, "Luis, there really never is going to be a Friday Night's Lights for you or your boys is there?" That caught me off guard a little, as it was not where I was expecting the conversation to go. I replied, "Probably not." After a short time he said, "I'm sorry. I never realized it. I'm so sorry you will not get a chance to enjoy that experience with your own boys." I responded that I was lucky in other ways with regard to my boys. No, I was never going to have that thrill, but Kyler and Koleden bring me a different and unique happiness that he will never get to enjoy with his boys.

CHAPTER FIFTEEN

To Medicate or Not To Medicate?

"He scares himself when his medication isn't working properly. He knows he's out of control; he just has no way of controlling himself."

"He has been taught right from wrong in many situations, but if it's a new situation, he has difficulty making that connection."

Although we did not know it at the time, the decision to try medications was a major turning point for us. I was resistant to the idea of giving or forcing my 6-year old son to take pills. I thought medication was for sick people, and my son was not sick!! Remember our two long-term main goals for Kyler? First we wanted him to have the ability to function in a mainstream classroom. Our second goal was to help him progress to the point that people just upon meeting him might find him a bit different, but they would not really know what was wrong with him. They would know he was just a little different if they paid attention. Well, neither of those goals were being achieved at the time.

We put him in a mainstream kindergarten, and even with special accommodations he just could not function. Kyler's behavior had improved dramatically over the past few years and he was pretty good in a lot of instances, but in situations with lots of external stimulation, like a classroom environment, he would literally start bouncing off the walls, screaming, hitting his head, or just shut down, at which point he could be a danger to himself or others. There was not a middle ground type of behavior. Autism was not yet hitting epidemic proportions and there was no roadmap for us or most mainstream teachers to follow. To say we were winging it concerning the school environment would be a fair statement. The one thing we knew was that book after book written up to that point stressed over and over again that it was our responsibility to be the advocate for our child. We could not wait for others to make decisions for us. We realized that teachers, administrators, and others in the public schools were not going to stand up for Kyler, so we had to do it. That was our job.

We wanted Kyler to be mainstreamed in school or at least to try it, but that was seeming more and more unlikely. Kyler had attended preschool from the age of three, but those were special needs programs. Our state provided an interventionist, Gayle, but the kindergarten teacher, as well as the site specialist in charge of Individual Education Plans (IEPs) told us that we would have to come up with other alternatives. Kyler just could not attend a mainstream class. He was disrupting the other students and he was not getting anything out of it himself. They suggested we see a psychiatrist. At that time I did not understand where things were going, but I was soon to find out. After meeting with a psychiatrist who specialized in working with children on the autism spectrum, she suggested a cocktail of medication. I was appalled at how much "crap" she wanted to shove down my son's throat. I was not okay with this!

Dana and I went home with very heavy hearts and concerns about what we were contemplating doing to our son. A conservative talk show host I sometime listened to would often rant and rave about how we were over medicating and destroying our children. His message was laced with disparaging remarks about parents who would subject their kids to those pill pushers. I have to admit I agreed to a large point with his thoughts. It seemed that people were too eager to turn to pharmaceutical companies to "fix" problems. I was not totally anti-medication but I wondered if such large doses were really needed to control kids? Couldn't most kids be controlled with better parenting skills? Was there more I should be doing as a father that could reverse the path Kyler was heading down? Questions and more questions came to mind but not a lot of answers.

After much soul searching and prayer, we decided to give the medication route a chance. Our goal was for Kyler to function in a mainstream classroom. We had been told that was not going to be possible without something else being done. We had to weigh the goal against the alternative which would have been to place him in special-ed classrooms for the rest of his life. We always pushed Kyler for more than what was expected, so we felt we had to at least give this a shot. At first we had only 2 or 3 very small pills which we had to teach him to swallow. One was shaped like a football so he called it the "football." For some reason Kyler had no problem trying that one. He was motivated to try that pill because he had played one year of youth football. The experience was a complete disaster, primarily due to his inability to comprehend one word the coaches said. He liked the idea of eating the football. We would hide the other pills in bananas or some soft food he did not have to chew. The results were not immediately fantastic, but we found that Kyler could focus a little more, bounced off the walls a little less, and generally was a little easier to teach. Every two weeks Dana took Kyler to the doctor for the new prescriptions (scripts) and a review of how the meds were working. Small subtle changes were made every visit until the doctor, the teacher, and Dana felt the cocktail was just right. Finally, they found just the right mix of medication that was a tremendous help to Kyler, his trainers, and teachers. We had reached our first goal; he was able to survive in a mainstream classroom if he had major accommodations and proper medication.

The medication made a big change in his life. He was a different kid, not a zombie as some people claim medication made kids. He was far less hyper and much more teachable.

So here I go on the first of many roller coaster rides thinking we found the "magic bullet" and Kyler was going to be cured!! I must admit that happened on numerous occasions in Kyler's youth. He would start to do things a little more on the normal side and I would think he was going to be all better. My hopes and dreams about my son would be realized and all those people that told me he had an incurable condition would be proven wrong. I now know I was just continuing in my denial and total lack of understanding of his neurological condition.

The benefits of the medical cocktail were not to last forever. As his body grew and his school environment changed from year to year, we found his need for differing quantities and types of medication would change. Thus we found another variable in the adjustments we were going to be constantly making to help Kyler find as full a life as possible.

Kyler taking a lot of medications can still be a bit of a struggle for me, but not how you think. Even now when we go out as a family, a full dosage of medications go with us. We never know when the occasion will arise that we will be out later than usual and he will need his night-time medication or his mid-day medication. We try to do this discreetly but sometimes he must take the pills in plain view of many people. It is literally a handful. I wonder if people are judging me, saying to themselves, "Look at all that crap those people are shoving down their kid's throats." Both my sons take 12 different medications throughout the day. I have come to worry less about what other people may think and worry more about how my boys are doing. How are they coping? Are they having a good time? Is the activity we are involved with enriching them?

Another situation that can be tough is sending the boys on an overnight campout with a church group. Two things have to happen. First: they must take their night-time meds or they will literally stay up all night. That can be convenient if we need them to stay up all night for a neurological exam the next morning, but it is not good if they are on a campout. Second: if they do not get their morning meds by 10:00 a.m. they are out of control for the rest of the day. In the event Kyler forgets to take his medication, he scares himself because he now realizes that he has considerably less control of his actions than he is used to. Without medication, Koleden will be so emotional that he will meltdown with tears or screams at the slightest provocation, real or imagined. Now here is the rub—we must explain to their church leaders the importance of their taking this boat load of medication. We must explain what happens if they don't take their meds, or what happens if they take the wrong ones, or what will happen if they lose them, etc.. Most people have never experienced Kyler off meds, but once they do they gain a new understanding of the condition he must deal with every day. These conditions have become easier for me to explain, but I still get a bit embarrassed and worry that people might still be judging me. I know from years of experience that what I'm doing is right for us, for me, but do others understand? I don't know, but it's a struggle that I will probably never totally overcome. It's a struggle that I will continually confront, but confront it I will. I'm doing it for my boys.

I could share story after story about the benefits of meds in Kyler's and Koleden's lives, but I will tell you just one more. One day in seventh grade Kyler forgot to take his morning meds before heading off to school. It was approaching 10:00 a.m. and he was starting to get out of control in the classroom. He started manifesting classic autistic traits that many of his classmates had never seen from Kyler. Over the course of an hour he started to hit his head on his desk, make strange baby noises, hit himself in the head with his hands, crawl under the desk, rock back and forth, etc.. The teacher was freaking out and did not know what to do. The school called my wife at home and on her cell, but there was no answer. They then called the first grade teacher, Mrs. Kathy, who had maintained a very close relationship with Kyler over the years. We held Kyler back in first grade and she developed a special relationship with him, so she had become the designated special-ed teacher at the school. That meant Mrs. Kathy knew him better than anyone else at the school. She knew exactly what had happened. Though it had been some time since she had seen that type of behavior from Kyler, she instantly knew the cause. Kyler had not taken his meds. She had him removed from the room so that he would not further disrupt the class, but also so that his classmates would not see or experience the real Kyler and develop a negative attitude or impression of him. That already existed to a point. They knew Kyler was different; they just did not know or understand how different. Mrs. Kathy knew there was medication at the school for just this situation, and she had Kyler under control within an hour. We were so blessed to have had such a supportive charter school where the staff actually cared about our son.

Although I am still not a fan of over-medicating our children in general, medication must play a major role in our boys' lives. Others will have to make their own decisions on whether medication is right for them. It is a very difficult decision which further makes parents wonder if it is their fault they sired a child who needs so many pills to function. Was this caused by my genes or WHAT? I know one thing: whatever the reason it happened, it does not matter. It did happen. All that matters now is how I must man-up and help my children to the best of my ability and resources. And if that is just to love them with all my heart, no matter the obstacles I must endure, then that's what I must do.

CHAPTER SIXTEEN

SIBLING ISSUES

"It makes me crazy when those around him who should be trying to understand what makes him tick just say he's normal and he's okay."

Many years ago an associate of mine who had grown up with a special needs brother gave me a very good piece of advice. She told me, "Do not forget about the needs of your other kids while investing so much time helping Kyler."

We have four children, two bookend girls with two autistic boys in the middle. Brenna, the oldest daughter, has had to deal with her own frustrations and rejections at the hands of others due to Kyler's condition.

Brenna and Kyler are just 17-months apart in age and should be only one grade apart in school. However, we held Kyler back in 1st grade to give him additional time to catch up with age appropriate students. There is a close overlap in friends, for Brenna more than for Kyler. The truth of the matter is that Kyler does not have many friends due to his weird ways and his general lack of maturity when being around teenagers his own age or slightly older. This affects Brenna when it comes to church and school friends.

There are some unwritten rules in those two areas. The one that seems to really come into play is getting invited to birthday parties or non-church related parties/get togethers. Kyler does not get his feelings hurt when not invited to social events or parties, but the non-invites often include Brenna. On a few occasions Brenna has found out that the only reason she was not invited to an event was because they did not want to include Kyler. So instead of just inviting Brenna, they didn't invite either. This has often been painful for her. She wants to be included, but she often is not. This frustrates me beyond what I want to admit. I want to call the parents of these offending kids and tell them to get a clue, to try and get them to understand our situation. We know Kyler is different; we know other kids do not want him around, but please don't take it out on Brenna. This situation goes for my son Koleden and his sister Shea as well. Often these people are friends of mine who just don't get it. I guess that is one of the reasons I started to write this book: to give a voice to the fathers out there who are experiencing the same things, feelings, or thoughts. I wanted to give them a way to communicate to others through a third party.

A solution we have found that has worked out well is to allow Brenna to be involved in activities outside of church and school. By doing this she has developed friendships and associations much removed from our regular sphere of influence. We have done everything we can to encourage this and allow her to develop these relationships: sleepovers, parties, extra events, etc.. This has created an environment where Kyler is not a consideration, because there is no built-in association. Brenna is able to cultivate those friendships and be fully included in activities with no repercussions because of Kyler.

When Kyler was diagnosed, he began to receive a lot of attention from adults—doctors, therapists, teachers, aids, the schools, and most of all his mother. Brenna, being the older sister, was not getting any of that. Dana was running the two kids around constantly, but Brenna was not getting any special attention. What was therapy to Kyler looked like fun play time to Brenna. Dana spent hours working with

Kyler on balls and swings and using sensory brushes. We did not know it, but we were causing Brenna a certain level of anxiety that caused a phobia of dogs to develop almost overnight. She couldn't take out her anxiety on her brother or her mother, so she manifested it on dogs, any dog. They could be puppies that were the size of a hand or huge mastiffs. She became deathly afraid of them. This lasted for years. She had been raised with our Queensland Healer and loved her, but she woke up one morning so afraid of our dog that she could not be in the same room. Our doctor explained that Brenna developed a resentment, not so much of Kyler and all the attention he was getting but a deep rooted resentment for the attention she was not getting. Naturally a certain level of jealousy existed and had to be manifested in some way, and a phobia of dogs was it.

These long held resentments Brenna has been carrying around have definitely extended into her teenage years. As odd as it may sound, even now as a teenager she sometimes will want her own time with her parents. She will ask for her own one-on-one time with her mom or me, even if it is just to go out and get an ice cream cone. Brenna is not a selfish person at all, but I think internally she must feel she did not get as much attention as she deserved. We tried to listen to my friend's advice, "do not forget about your other kids," but in the end I don't think we did a very good job.

A strange dynamic that developed was the relationship between our youngest daughter, Shea, and Brenna. It truly is amazing how much they love each other. They play together, eat popcorn and watch movies, or just enjoy being in the car listening to blarring music together. This said, Brenna can be very jealous of any extra attention we give to her little sister. Brenna has a hard time seeing any attention going Shea's way. Shea idolizes Brenna and wants to please her. As we move on through life, I hope and pray they will hold on to the love they share and not the jealousy they may feel because they did not get the attention from their parents that their brothers did.

This of course leaves me once again beating myself up for not being the perfect dad and for not giving enough of myself to my wonderful girls. It seems I can be angry "at me" for another failed part of my parenting.

I can be greatful for some assistance as it relates to Brenna's upbringing. Brenna developed a special relationship with her maternal grandparents, and they have been more than happy to reciprocate. This is a relationship only she has, and she loves it. It makes her feel special. I guess I could be jealous of this situation, but I am not. I know it is good for Brenna and that is enough.

CHAPTER SEVENTEEN

MACHISMOISM

"It makes me extremely angry when people tell me Kyler can do something, but he just doesn't want to."

"He's cried in my arms because he doesn't understand why nobody wants to be around him."

We, okay I, went through a tough patch with Brenna when she was in 4th and 5th grades. She became hard for me to control. That should tell you everything about me right there. I felt I had to control everything and everyone in my sphere. She started to act up in school. Her grades started to suffer as she made little or no attempt to do a good job. She would not obey at home and would defy me at all possible opportunities. She would go out of her way to make belittling comments to me in public. I was not okay with that in any way, shape, or form. I was at my wits end, and we often would go days without talking. It even came to the point where I considered letting her move in with her grandparents. I just could not personally deal with such a disruptive child. I even spent some time with a friend who is a therapist. This of course came after many months of denial that I was in any way part of the problem.

I was raised in a culture where "children are seen and not heard," and the male ruled the home and was not questioned by the children. To have my young daughter not fit into this mold caused me a lot of boiling frustration and anger. The prevailing message that I was getting from my wife and the therapist was that I was the parent. I was the adult and many of my actions were that of a child. We were not raising a family based on the machismo attitude of my youth. I had to keep reminding myself of that. However, I was the male and it was hard for me to accept because I *felt* I was the parent. I was the bread winner. I was the adult. Therefore, I *should* be in charge. I finally realized that was not going to work in my situation. Now I did not, nor have I come to believe, that my daughter and I are equals. I still have all the above roles, but I am no longer the dictator of my family and home. I guess I could go on for pages about this, but let me cut to the chase. It took lots of patience and coaching on my wife's part, and a fair amount of re-education on my part, to understand that I was the adult/parent (not a dictator) and needed to start acting like one. I lost those years with my oldest daughter, but over time I began to repair my relationship with her. I feel the past 4-5 years have been a wonderful rediscovery of each other. Building our friendship has been a great experience. I have also come to understand that I was not the only one dealing with the difficulty of having a son with a disability, but my daughter was dealing on a daily, no hourly basis, with the needs and attention of an autistic brother. Her pain was equal, if not more, than mine since peer pressure plays such a major role in kids' lives.

I have had to put aside my machismo background and look at myself and what I can do to improve my weaknesses. I was so determined to control everyone that I was unable to see anyone (Brenna) else's opinion. Everyone in my family is affected by autism, not just me.

CHAPTER EIGHTEEN
FAMILY DENIAL

"It's frustrating when people who are with him for a long time finally have the light go on, and they understand that he's just not in there, but they could've made such a difference if they had just listened in the first place."

It is so discouraging when our families tell us Kyler's fine; he's normal; he's just a boy; he's a second child; there is nothing wrong with him. Three thoughts here. One, I'm glad we did not listen to them then or now. Two, I cannot believe not one person on either side of our families researched and tried to learn about autism. Three, it's amazing how very little some of them understand Kyler and Koleden and the life we live with them even to this day when Kyler is 16 years of age and Koleden is 13.

I have been told by a relative in the past year or so that there is nothing wrong with Kyler; he's fine; he's catching up; don't know what all the fuss was about. That has been this relative's line for the past 15 years!!!! I wish he could walk in my shoes for one week, through the melt downs, through the mood swings, through the depression, through the special diets, the doctor's appointments, the multiple therapy sessions, the psychiatrist's visits, the multiple visits to the pharmacy that can sometimes take an entire day, the self-mutilation, the emotional abuse, the bullies, the IEP sessions at the schools, the teachers at schools demanding he keep up in their class rooms, the teacher telling our daughter that autism is caused by moms who are refrigerator moms, throughout the frustration of it all. Then, maybe, they would have a small inkling of what my family has been going through for the past 15 years, month after grinding month, and year after year. Worse—we have it two-fold since we have two boys with autism, and we hear the same thing for both of them.

One day Kyler was struggling to self-monitor himself. He was acting anti-social (moody), when some family came by unannounced. A cousin noticed his non-friendly behavior and asked his parent, "What's wrong with Kyler?" The parent retorted with an off handed remark of, "Oh just ignore him. He's in one of his moods." His moods?!!! Are you freaking kidding me? How about saying, "Kyler is struggling with how to act today. Why don't you see if you can cheer him up?" or "Maybe you can help Kyler feel better, if you see what he wants to do and help him do it." Sometimes family members say things that just hurt, not meaning to, but hurt none-the-less.

Kyler has been aware for some time that he needs to take his medication, otherwise he cannot control himself. On occasions when he is out of control and I try to discuss what he is feeling and why he is doing crazy things, his responses are very interesting. He has shared in these instances that he scares himself due to his lack of control over his own actions. He knows what he is doing is wrong, but he can't stop himself. Often times, even on medication, he just can't manage his feelings and emotions. This worries him and causes him compounded concern because he does not know what he may do next. As his father, this is doubly worrisome. I fear that he might hurt someone in a rage. Will he hurt himself in such a way that there is no returning from his action? His safety and the safety of others are always concerns. Up to this point he has not done anything too alarming, but what is he capable of now that he is larger and stronger? I just don't know, and it scares me. He has had intensive training since the age of two and is *unusually* self-aware.

He may not be able to control it, but he knows when his system is out of alignment.

Since Kyler became aware of his condition, he has said things like, "I don't want to be autistic anymore" or "When I go to heaven will I still have to be autistic?" He has even said, "I wish I were dead so that I wouldn't be autistic anymore." These statements cause an emotional strain on me from the pit of my stomach to the back of my throat. I almost want to cry. In fact, I do cry a little on the inside. He does not want to be like he is, but other than Dana, Brenna, and I, others around us just don't understand. I guess they can't, but it would be so much easier on us if others understood. If they could know how to help him, help us, by being understanding and not dismissive. We would have thought/hoped that family members would have tried to educate themselves a little on autism so that they could support us. It did not happen for us, but when we talk to families who have been newly diagnosed we stress the importance of this support.

We are lucky in that we have found or had placed in our lives many wonderful professionals who do understand what we are going through. They have validated our concerns, worries, fears, helplessness, and despair. When no one else could support us in our times of concern, they could and did. They knew the right words and helped us find ways to deal with everything. Sometimes all they did was offer a shoulder to lean on, but sometimes that's all I needed. They gave me that little extra boost to get me through the day so that I could face the next hurdle, so that I could get up once more from my fallen state and try to "Win the race!"

CHAPTER NINETEEN

MY SECOND SON, MY SECOND CHANCE!

"Why do people think I'm just making excuses for my son when I try to explain to them a little bit about him? Since when are they the experts just because he looks normal and should act normal? They're surprised when they finally come to learn that he is not the same as every other kid. This frustrates me to no end because so much could have been done to help him have a positive experience, but they have come to this knowledge far too late."

I know I have already mentioned my second son Koleden, but I want to give a little added information to this entire episode and how I dealt with it. Dana was again pregnant. At that time Kyler was 2 1/2 and involved with several kinds of therapies multiple times a week, and the full impact of his development and his future life was still shrouded in a fog of uncertainty. I also had in no way started to come to terms with his autism. This said, my second son was on the way. I had a second chance at a boy who could be the standard bearer for me and the family, my family name. As I have mentioned before in great detail, my hopes, dreams, and expectations were even more enhanced for MY second son. He is gonna fill the void that will be left by Kyler. I could not have been more excited and filled with expectations. Koleden's birth was not nearly the scary event of Kyler's. The baby was doing well until the very end. He was coming down the birth canal with the umbilical cord tightening around his neck, cutting down on his oxygen intake. The doctor worked quickly and cut the cord before he was even out and born.

They put him on oxygen, and his APGAR scores fell well within the normal range. The comment kept going around that they had never seen such a healthy and pliable umbilical cord. That was the reason that he showed no signs of distress during the labor process.

Koleden's early life development was close to right on track. He was able to meet all the standard milestones in successive appointments with his pediatrician. As an infant he did have an issue with metatarsus adductus. His outer foot bones were curved like a C toward his big toe. We met with a podiatrist and he prescribed a special shoe for his foot. Koleden had to wear that ugly shoe for over a year, but with time his foot straightened out, and he continued his normal development, both physically and mentally. As a small child he was hyper-focused on trains. He could create the most elaborate train sets down to the most minute detail. Koleden was a happy child, very engaging with a quick smile and a laugh. To see him and interact with him was a joy. He was also growing quickly, ranking at the 100 percentile in height and over 90 percentile in weight. He was going to be my big boy. All a dad's dreams of the future for my boys was going to fall to Koleden.

Kyler was born with autism and had very clear signs of it from the time he was an infant; Koleden was different. He was as normal as could be as he was exiting the toddler stage and developing a real personality. At the age of 18-months he did need some speech therapy until the age of three, but nothing serious, so we thought. Around the age of 5 everything started to go very wrong. Late-onset-autism is an event that happens both quickly (on the calendar) and slowly (as you witness it) at the same time. Kids who were perfectly normal stop smiling, stop interacting with other kids or adults, stop making eye contact, stop eating the foods they loved just a month before, stop talking, etc.. Those are just phrases and comments, but unless you live it you cannot comprehend it. You cannot know the utter helplessness and hopelessness you feel watching your child slip away to a shell of his previous self.

I don't know how to relate it to a normal person, but I'll throw an idea out and see if it makes sense. Think of a person losing his sight gradually over the course of several months from macular degeneration. He can see it happening. He may notice the differences every day but can do nothing to stop it. Then one day he wakes up and he is blind. It's like the light was just slowly turned off and now it's all gone. Watching your child's light go out is not much different. From one month to another the light slowly goes out and you're left very scared, alone, angry, confused, lost, and desperate to find answers. But there are none. Your child has slipped away into the dumbfounding world of autism.

For those who have lived this nightmare, it's crushing. For those who have not, it's viewed as sad or unfortunate. What it most definitely is, is a life changing event that will never leave you the same.

Kyler, our first son, was 8-years old and moving slowly, ever slowly, through his development with massive amounts of therapy and medication. We were still ill-equipped to deal with the issues surrounding Koleden's developmental issues. His situation was new to us, even though he was falling into the world of autism, a world we were starting to become familiar with, we did not recognize it or see it coming in Koleden's case.

Koleden was due to start school at 5 1/2-years of age like all other children. When Dana went to register him for school, the administrator noted that he was not totally up to date on all his inoculations. We had put off giving him his MMR (Measles, Mumps, & Rubella). According to the school, this was required for him to attend. (We have learned differently and never had our youngest daughter Shea inoculated). So Dana made an appointment with Koleden's pediatrician. The visit went like clockwork; his development was good and he was given his final shots, including the MMR, so he could enter school.

Koleden had been so normal, generally so on track, that what was happening to him, his odd behavior, had to be a phase. I had become rigidly attached to the fact that he was going to be the boy I had always wanted. He was going to fulfill all the dreams that Kyler could not. For months Koleden regressed and for months I did not see it. I became very impatient with him for not understanding. I did not want to accept what was happening. With Kyler it had been different. He was always behind, different, quirky, so classically autistic from the beginning that it allowed me to slowly wrap my head around it. I was able to come to terms with it over a long period of time.

Koleden was different. His development had only the one official hiccup and because of our large network of therapists for Kyler, we were able to get Koleden immediate help. At 18-months, Koleden was diagnosed as slightly speech delayed. So we took him to see Kyler's speech therapist, Louise. She primarily worked with autistic kids but was happy to assist us with Koleden. After 18 months of therapy she declared Koleden age appropriate in speech and language. We were on our way. During Koleden's youth he would often attend Kyler's occupational therapy sessions, interacting with him and his therapists.

The next few months would change our lives forever. That was when Koleden's regression began. We missed all the clues of late onset autism because we were in denial about what was happening. We chalked up his regression to the transition of going to school and stress by being separated from his mom and his little sister,

Shea. These two played together like two little bear cubs. They are 18-months apart and they loved each other.

He started to change right under our noses. He lost language, stopped making eye contact, and his appetite was dwindling. He started to lose weight at an alarming rate. By October, the school called my wife in for a consultation about Koleden. The school psychologist, unbeknownst to us, had been doing some testing with him. She shared with my wife that she thought Koleden's behavior and learning difficulties indicated he might fall on the high end of the autistic spectrum, possibly Asperger's Syndrome. My wife was crying when she called me, and we were on the road to find out what was happening to our (my) perfect little son. But more than that, I had to find out if the dreams I had for my boy were going to be dashed once more.

My wife started the rounds of multiple doctors, psychologists, psychiatrists, neurologists, speech therapists, occupational therapists, physical therapists. We placed Koleden in a study at the University of Arizona headed by a top neurological doctor in autism research. By January we had the official news. Koleden was on the autism spectrum. When we took Koleden back to his speech therapist and Kyler's occupational therapist, they were shocked at how much Koleden had changed over the past 24 months. They had worked with Koleden at length and were experts working with autistic children, and to see how Koleden had changed caught them off guard. They could not believe it was the same child.

My world was once again shattered. My fatherly hopes for my second son gone. I now reflect on how I behaved during that period of our life and am somewhat ashamed. I was clearly in denial during Koleden's slide into the world of autism. As Koleden was regressing, my patience with his developing strange behaviors made me angry. I did not show him the love and compassion he needed.

Instead, I expected him to be more, to do more, to speak more, to act NORMAL. As his behaviors became more annoying to his sisters, I did not hesitate to punish him with a swat or grounding him to his room. My patience with him while teaching him golf and baseball was nearly nothing. When working with him on his school work I found myself unable to deal with his lack of focus or comprehension. His tantrums were driving me nuts, which led to more swats and room punishments. I know now my wife and daughters were going through the same thing, but I just could not face it. I know my wife was crushed with the news of a second autistic son and I left her to pick up the pieces. I reflect back on those times with a certain amount of self loathing, but how was I supposed to act? Looking back at it I know I could have and should have handled it better, but I still struggle with how or what I should have done differently. I know I should have, but....I was so confused, crushed and in continual denial that I did not know what to do. My heart aches for that time in my life and the pain I left my family in. I am so blessed they stayed with me.

CHAPTER TWENTY

TIPPING POINT & MARRIAGE

*"He's quiet and therefore not disruptive, so people
conclude there is nothing wrong with him. He's quiet
because the world is just 'Noise' to him."*

A crazy statistic is available regarding the number of fathers who just can't stand by their families during this very difficult journey. According to stats from the National Institute of Health, 2011: (*www.ncbi.nlm.nih.gov/pmc/articles/PMC2928572/*) concerning parents of special needs children, between 80-90% of married couples who have special needs kids end in divorce. That is a staggering number. It is also scary. It takes a lot of effort on both sides to keep the marriage alive. One thing we heard, which I believe is true, is that "special needs children must have parents with special marriages." There must be communication on both sides. At the time of Kyler's diagnosis in 1999, the odds of autism were 1 in 1,000. As of 2014, the CDC announced the odds are 1 in 68.

Koleden's diagnosis was a tipping point in our lives. Which way would our lives, our marriage, my family tip? This period marked a point in our lives that would prove to be the big crossroad, the proverbial "Y" in the road. Our marriage was struggling or better said—I was not trying to make our marriage work. I became despondent and withdrawn. I may have lived at home but it was just a place to live, to sleep, and to eat. I was not treating it like a home, and I turned even more to my work, 13-15 hour days with only Sundays off. I would go to church, then go home and sleep the rest of the day. I lived like a zombie, not feeling much, not enjoying much, not giving much of myself to my family.

Dana was getting more and more frustrated with me for my lack of being a good understanding dad. She was angry with how I could show so much patience with Kyler and almost none for Koleden. Even though we did not know what was going on with that second son, she could clearly see I was losing it with him, with my boy. I was lucky I had work, and I buried myself in it. Owning my own struggling small business gave me the excuse to spend more time away from home and the world that was crashing down around me. At work I was able to control my surroundings and the tasks that needed to be completed. That was not the case at home. I spent more and more time at work and less at home.

I never even thought about my poor wife who was the one who had to face the problems that another child with autism represented. She was the one who had to go to all the specialists and make all the appointments and get all the meds. She was the one who had to do home therapy with the boys as well as take care of the girls and the house and the bills. She had to advocate for the boys at school and had to hold our family together emotionally because I was unable to face my life at this time. She was a single mom without it being official. Our interventionist was surprised that we had not asked for either of our boy's to be placed in special homes available for autistic people. Every time she came to the house she would remind us of that option at the end of each visit.

My incredible wife single-handedly saved our marriage. Many times that same interventionist would remark how amazed she was that we were still married. I wish I could have responded that it was because both my wife and I worked really hard at it, but I couldn't say that. I was in such a state of depression that I could not see that my wife was single-handedly holding the family together, but she was tired. She has a childhood friend, Jodi, who is a psychologist, and my wife suggested that I talk with her, but I was way too proud to consider counseling. I was okay; there was nothing wrong with me. I told myself I was a good father and husband because I went to work and provided for my family. My work allowed my wife to stay home and raise our children. What else was I truly responsible for? That was how I was raised. That was what I saw my dad do, so why did I have to do more? That would prove to be a dark time in my family's life.

On the outside looking in, everyone I knew thought I was dealing remarkably well with what was going on in my life. On the inside, I was wondering how to run away and stop the disappointment that was a constant barrage in my life. On many occasions my wife would say to me "We need to talk." That was code to me that I was in trouble. She would do her best trying to help me see what I was doing, how I was acting. She was trying to understand what was happening to me, but I could not see it, especially at first. I was defensive and unwilling to listen to her. I felt she could not understand what I was feeling or going through. "What was I thinking?"

As I look back I am truly amazed that she stayed with me and fought for our family. Finally, she suggested I try an herbal remedy called *Sam-e* that could help me with my ever-changing mood swings (undiagnosed depression). She also got me to speak with a professional about what I was going through. She told me she was thinking of moving out, and I was angry at her. How dare she threaten that! I was doing everything.....wait, maybe she was right. I loved my family and did not want to lose them, especially if it might actually be my fault. I was not ready at that point to admit that it was me. So I consented to speak over the phone to her psychologist friend, Jodi, and be open-minded about the process. That was my first step to overcoming the baggage I was holding onto from my childhood that was preventing me from growing as a person. I looked to find where I could grow as a husband, father, friend, and contributor to our family beyond being the financial supporter. I read books then I talked about what I read with my wife and recognized/identified many of the difficulties I was struggling with were from deep seeded insecurities from my past.

Looking back, there is no question in my mind I had issues, but to admit it was not going to happen quickly. I had to change on my own, one step at a time, one day at a time, one example at a time. My wife and I have learned to have many discussions and exchanging of ideas and perspectives about our family. I have also had to admit that I was not always right. I have had to let go of the machismo attitude I was raised on, so that I could have my family and appreciate my boys.

Another casualty of that time of my life was my wonderful daughter Brenna. As the oldest, I had already transferred onto her the need to be far older than she was, more responsible in every sense of the word. I wanted her to help her mother at home with the kids and all household duties. Kyler was already wearing us out and we were looking for answers about what was happening to Koleden. I would often take Brenna to work on the weekends and would expect a 9-year old to keep up with me. What the heck was I thinking? That was not only unfair but damaging to our relationship—damage that has taken years to begin to repair. I fear it will take many years (maybe never) to repair the harm that came from my not being able to control my emotions and frustrations during that time of my life. However, I will never stop trying.

Over the course of the last few years many things came together for me. The first and most important thing was to come to appreciate my wife and become familiar with her struggles. What I was going through was not just happening to me. She was the one in the trenches. She was the one who had to deal with the problems 24/7. I escaped to my work for 12-15 hours a day. She was the one who had to deal with all the professionals and therapists who worked with the boys. She was the one who had to deal with all the appointments and medication changes. She was the one who had to advocate at the school and with the teachers. Love between parents can make all the harder trials in life a little easier. My wife saved our marriage, but I had to let it be saved, and for a proud man who was not in control of his life, that was not easy. I had to let my love for my family trump all other feelings. My family is what makes my life full and complete. Without them, my life would be lonely and empty.

Second, my daughters are a sacred gift to me from my Heavenly Father. Treating them as anything less is not acceptable. They are living this difficult life with us and having two autistic brothers is no picnic. Making sure they know they are special and important has been crucial. Every day I tell them I love them and am proud of them. They are amazing young ladies and deserve to be treated as such.

Finally, my boys need to be raised by a mom AND a dad. They will progress to the point they can. No one knows what that means, but I have to help them get there. Now I take joy from this prospect and from this journey. Their love is unconditional and most likely always will be, not because I'm their dad but because I love them for who they are.

I will never be done growing as a person; I must continually keep working to become a better husband, father, and friend, to the most important people in my life—My Family.

The importance of balance in work, family, and religion has not come easy for me to accomplish, but when these three things come into balance so do many of the other things in life.

My faith in God is a driving force for me. I knew what I wanted in my life spiritually but sometimes found it hard considering the difficulty I was having coping with my boys' lifetime disabilities. I've held tight to our religious beliefs regarding families and perfection after this life, and it provides me strength. Life throws us curves and the question we have to ask ourselves is: Are we going to bail out in fear, or are we going to stay in the game, watch the ball, and swing for the fences? If you don't swing you will never hit the ball. If you don't stay in there regardless of the fear you feel, you will never experience the thrill of getting good wood on the ball. If you don't get up each time you fall, you will never know the pride of finishing the race. The same applies to the experience of raising autistic children. Fear, failure, and uncertainty will accompany your journey, but moments of thrill will be even sweeter when they happen. Enjoy the journey, love the challenges, bask in the success. It will not always be easy but your marriage and family will always be worth it.

CHAPTER TWENTY ONE
FEEDING TUBES?

*"As a young toddler he was malnutritioned and many
doctors said he'll eat when he's hungry. One specialist
said, 'He doesn't know that he's hungry. He doesn't know
he is starving. He doesn't know that he's killing himself.
He doesn't understand that without food he will die.'
Doctors don't even know what to do with him."*

Both the boys have been clinically diagnosed with malnutrition at
some point in their early lives. I now look at those events and know
I was a big contributor to their condition. Being raised with the
age-old adage of "You'll eat what I put in front of you," and "A child
will eat once he is hungry enough" just did not apply to my boys, no
matter how hard I wanted it to be true. Unfortunately, that did not
become clear to me for many years. After much reflection I realize it
was my continued denial of their condition that caused the problem.

Both boys came out of their first 18 months of life being on the high
end of the age appropriate scale in weight and height. That was
as it should be if they were going to fulfill my personal dreams for
my boys. Around the age of 5 the weight started to fall off, and in
Koleden's case at an alarming rate. Koleden went from near the 100
percentile in weight down to the 20 percentile in just over a year.
Once it had been decided that he was now clinically malnutritioned
the pediatrician sent us to a Pediatric Gastroenterologist to see if
there was something going on in his system that was causing this
to happen. I wondered if he might have tapeworms or some other

strange digestive issue. I knew he was not eating much, but I was not home often. I truly believed that no kid would starve himself. The Pediatric Gastroenterologist had an easy solution to the problem once we had ruled out any weird or strange intestinal problems. The doctor suggested we should have feeding tubes surgically placed in Koleden's body, and we could feed him through a tube. Now I was generally all for listening to the doctors and their professional advice but a "feeding tube"? That seemed a bit of an extreme and over the top solution. I was not going to put a tube in my boy so we could feed him with a syringe for the rest of his life. He was not going to be some freak at school feeding himself with a tube. This was not going to happen, and I was not happy with that option.

So we went looking for another possible solution. We tried a nutritionist who specialized in special needs kids. She did a rather long interview where she tried to understand Koleden's eating habits and what he liked and disliked. She made a rather strange declaration: "Let him eat ice cream and as much of it as he wants." She said to allow him to eat all the strawberries with sugar he wanted and to put extra butter on his pancakes. I was absolutely stunned. We all like ice cream, strawberries, and pancakes, but a steady diet of those things could not be good for him or us. She also told us to let him eat any other sweets he wanted. That was a nutritionist saying those things—a person who is supposed to help us eat more healthy and direct us to consume more fruits and vegetables. Was I hearing her right? I even had to repeat her suggestions several times because I truly could not believe what she was saying. The words all made sense, but the message was all wrong. She said he needed calories, however unhealthy we may believe them to be. Otherwise he would just continue to starve himself. At that point he was truly skin and bones.

So I left a bit dumfounded, but I was willing to try that solution other than the option of the feeding tube, which I was not willing to try. And so began the unhealthy eating habits of my son. At first, okay for a very long time, okay still to this day, it is difficult for me to watch what my boys eat. The malnutrition issues are gone. In fact Koleden is now a bit on the heavy side, but that is better than the alternative. I am constantly aware of the boys' eating habits, such as the grazing, portions, late eating times, kind of calories, etc.. Now that they are older, I am even able to get them to try some foods I eat, even if it is just a bite. Sometimes on very rare occasions they will even like what they are trying. But always, in the end, they want to return to the safe foods they know best. When I barbecue, I have to make sure I do not allow any of the meat to blacken or get crunchy. Sometimes I'll make a nice meal and all they will eat are the mashed potatoes, no lumps. I could go on and on about the foods they won't eat, but what I have mostly come to terms with is that they will eat what they like (taste or texture) or they will go hungry. We try to keep what little fruit they will eat in the house. Vegetables? Well, they are vegetables so I guess that goes without saying—they are crunchy so they are out. Sugared cereals, not what I want them eating, but they will eat them so I try to ignore it. Soft pancakes and spaghetti with plain sauce could be on the menu 7 days a week and that would be just fine with them. So we now eat whatever we eat and if the boys want something off their food wheel, then that's what they will have, however crazy it sometimes makes me. I have learned over the long haul that is not a battle I will win.

CHAPTER TWENTY TWO
THE IEP: INDIVIDUAL EDUCATION PLAN

"To him you're speaking a foreign language. He just doesn't understand."

Ask any father of an ASD (Autism Spectrum Disorder) child about his IEP (Individual Education Plan) and watch his face contort right in front of your eyes. That is the most frustrating, maddening, and contentious meeting I have ever had the misfortune to attend. And here is the kicker: I now have to attend them multiple times a year. In the beginning I did attend the first few of those meetings but I just could not handle the constant platitudes and lack of progress. I did not want to rock the boat with the school, as I was sure they were doing all they could, so I left it to my wife to attend. I had to go to work and provide for the family. My wife had been a school teacher, so she could handle that stuff better. What I have come to learn is that it takes a team of professionals and two parents to take on the team of teachers and administrators across the table at the IEP.

As a father of an ASD child, I know his strengths and weaknesses. I understand/know his quirks. I see his melt downs from overwork or over-stimulation. I'm not fooling myself, I know who he is. So when I enter the IEP I know what my child is capable of and I find it absolutely astounding that all the people in the room who spend hundreds of hours a year with him still do not understand much about him. In some cases they know NOTHING ABOUT HIM.

They are supposed to be professional educators, but it sometimes seems like some are just there to collect their check.

We now know that all ASD kids are unique and different; each falls on the very large ASD spectrum with little idiosyncrasies that are unique to them. Although many ASD kids have similar traits, they don't fit a nice little package of learning and coping abilities. Although the same can be said for normal kids, it is in no way similar.

Schools are required by law to educate ASD kids, not to the best of their abilities, but to the standards set forth by the IEP. But how does this work? Who is responsible? How is it measured? Who keeps tabs? Who?..., What?..., Where is the end? As the parent of my boys, it is my job to see that all that gets done, that my boys are pushed to be all they can be, so that their education will help them become useful members of society. When dealing with schools, it often seems their goal is to get children passed through the system with as little effort as possible. That may seem a bit harsh, but I have never come out of an IEP meeting feeling like the school was doing everything in its power to mesh what we were doing outside of the school to improve the development of my boys. Every school is different even in the same school district. Some schools have better trained teachers, counselors, advocates, and principals.

Every IEP I have attended has a few components that are the same. The educators telling us how well the child is doing, a written plan of specific goals they would like to achieve academically, and some accommodations they are going to make to assist in making the kid's life a little bit easier. Sounds nice doesn't it? But what I have always found is that the expectations are always woefully low; the mental well-being of the child is not always met; the physical health and emotional needs of the child may not be considered, and the school is oblivious as to how my boy's daily interactions with students and teachers are causing him mental/physical anguish day after day. They are there with him. How are they not seeing those things? How can they be so clueless? How can they not see what is happening to him on a daily basis? I'm home with him at most 3 hours a day and I can see the damage being done to him at school, and they're not seeing any of it in 7 hours? If they are witnessing it, why are they waiting for the IEP to try and get this stuff worked out? Why must the parents be the ones to initiate all contact with the school, only after the damage is being done to my child? Why? Why? Why?

So how have we made the IEP work for us? In the beginning we would bring along an advocate from the state. Some districts have advocates for special needs kids. These advocates' sole responsibility is to help parents hold the school responsible/accountable for their child's education. They know the right phrases, catch words, and what seems like outlandish accommodations which need to be made to assist a special needs child. We have on occasion had to bring in professionals to help us get our message across as to our concerns and our desired educational goals.

As a parent entering an IEP, balancing the needs of your child with not wanting to alienate the people at the school seems like an impossible task. In some cases it is, but I have learned to attend the IEP with my desired goals, and if something does not seem right, then I question it. If the teachers are not giving my child what he needs, then I demand it. I have not yet had to go the legal route to get what I need for my boys. I guess I am lucky in that regard. I just wish I had been more involved in the process when they were younger.

CHAPTER TWENTY THREE
How They Crack Us Up!

Kyler's favorite subject in school is P.E. where he gets to play all types of sports. He came home one day and said, "Dad, I hate soccer!" "Why?" I asked. "I don't know what to do. I'm terrible. My feet are too far away from my brain."

"I'm a <u>MAN</u>, I have armpit hair!"

I have talked about negatives and hardships but there are also such funny and happy moments in my life. Having my boys with autism can just sometimes be so much fun. They do and say things that are so out there; all I can do is bust up laughing. I guess those are the rewards for becoming parents and taking on the responsibilities of rearing children. When you have kids with special needs, the good times just seem to stick out so much more. Koleden is extremely literal, so we have to be careful what we say. Kyler is literal but not to that extent. His big problem is how he comprehends what is said. Here are some examples that have just always made us laugh. I hope they give you an insight to the mind of an autistic child, but remember that every autistic child is different.

Fast Sunday
As members of The Church of Jesus Christ of Latter-day Saints, we fast for two meals on the first Sunday of each month and give the money we did not spend on food to the poor and needy. We believe that through this fast and prayer we can come closer to our Heavenly

Father and Jesus Christ. So, as with most months, we prepared as a family for our fast with prayer. I went up to my room to get ready for church. I came downstairs and my 8-year old son, Koleden, was moving through a bowl of cereal very quickly. I asked if he had forgotten it was Fast Sunday. He replied, with a mouth full of cereal and not slowing down, not missing a beat, in a voice indicating don't you know Dad, "It's FAST Sunday, and I got ready FAST and now I'm eating breakfast FAST!" "Literal" took on a whole new meaning for us.

Little League

As a former college baseball player I wanted to expose my sons to the national pastime. So from an early age, playing catch or teaching my boys to hit a ball in the back yard was one of our family activities. Little League, of course, was an activity my sons would participate in. One experience that was funny took place on the diamond. My younger son Koleden was in his second year of playing Minor ball. He had not had a hit yet and had not been swinging the bat in a game. So in preparation for the next game, we worked at taking that hard practice swing and using it in a game. I was coaching 1st base at the next game and was encouraging Koleden to swing at any pitch that was close. The first pitch went by and Koleden stepped out of the box and made a weak swing—"strike one." I called out encouragement to Koleden and repeated the need to swing hard to have a chance to hit the ball. A couple more pitches later and he continued to step back when the pitch went by. I was getting a bit frustrated at that point. I gave more encouragement and positive feedback to stay in there and swing the bat. The count was now 2 balls and 1 strike, and another pitch went by. Koleden still stepped back and made a weak swing. "Strike 2," was called by the umpire! I called from the coaching box, more than a little frustrated, "Koleden, did you lose your swing?" At that point Koleden stepped back and looked around the batter's box and the general area around him, appearing very confused. He then turned to his mom, who was seated behind the fence video taping, and said, "Where's my swing? I can't find it; I think I lost it!" Of course that cracked us up because of his literal thinking pattern. He truly thought he had lost his baseball swing.

Purse
Here is one that has happened a few times over the years. We were attending a wedding in southern California of one of my cousins. My sister was sitting on a small retaining wall in a beautiful garden area with Koleden sitting close by her. She needed to leave to get something to drink, so she asked Koleden to watch her purse. I was fairly close by but did not hear the exchange between the two. My sister left to do whatever she needed to do and returned to the area after a few minutes. When she got back, she noticed Koleden very intently staring at her purse. She innocently asked Koleden what he was doing? Without skipping a beat he replied, "I'm watching your purse!" That really caught her off guard and she came right over to me and related the story; she could not stop laughing.

Foreign Language
My father was born and raised in Mexico. He came to the United States at about the age of 15, but he still retains a strong accent. I was working one day and had to miss our weekly father/son baseball practice. My dad decided to take the boys out for a bit of practice. After some time on the field, my dad started to get a little frustrated with the boys because they were not following his directions. Following the next exchange my father came to understand why the boys were not following any of his instructions. After a short time, Kyler turned to my father and asked him, "Tata, why do you keep speaking to us in Spanish?" This caught him off gaurd and really made my dad start laughing to the point of crying, because he was speaking English the entire time.

We try to tell people that the boys understand about 25% of what is being said to them. Hearing someone speak in a unique or foreign accent changed their comprehension to near zero. In fact, knowing that my father also spoke Spanish as well as English, they assumed since they could not understand what he was telling them that he must be speaking Spanish. To this day if you ask my dad to relate that story he always laughs so hard he will start to tear up.

Gas Attendant

When Kyler was 15-years-old we were driving around town getting some errands done. We stopped by a convenience store to get some gas. I needed to go into the store to leave my credit card so I could fill up the truck. With Kyler in tow I went into the store. After giving the attendant my credit card I asked if he needed anything else. He quickly responded, "Yeah, your kid as a deposit as well." I smiled and said, "Thanks," and started to head out to the gas pump. I went through the front glass doors and turned to say something to Kyler. I didn't see him, so I glanced back into the store, and there was Kyler, dutifully standing at the counter as he felt instructed to do by the gas attendant. I walked back in and told Kyler he could come with me. He looked at me with a confused stare and said, "But he, (the attendant) wanted me to stay here." The attendant, a quick witted guy, realized what was going on and told Kyler it was okay for him to go with me. So out we went and off on our way. As I was lightly laughing at the situation I had to explain to a very confused Kyler why it was funny and how it was a saying commonly used by adults. He was still confused by the comment after several explanations, so I just left it. Kyler does not understand humor since he rarely understands entire conversations.

2 for 1

My wife was walking out of a major store that checked her receipt against what she had in her basket. Our youngest daughter, Shea, was riding underneath. The lady told my wife that she was unaware that they sold such beautiful little girls there at the store and that she would need to go check for more. Kyler was also walking out with my wife and the lady looked at him and said, "Oh, is it two for one day? I really must go back to get such beautiful children." As they left, Kyler turned to my wife and asked how she was going to go get more of them. Was it really a two for one child day? My wife just smiled and tried to explain that it was a joke. He was puzzled but did not get too upset.

As you can see, our life is not all negatives. It is actually quite fun now that I have come to accept the disability. It has taken me over 10 years of struggles, but I can say I am so happy to have my boys. I have something most dads will never have. I have sons who will consider me their hero forever. I have sons who might live with me the rest of their lives and bring me joy. I have sons who truly love me. I have had to change a lot. I have had to do a lot of soul searching and a lot of re-educating myself so that I am the man worthy of my family. I have two beautiful daughters, an angel for a wife, and two awesome sons. What more could I want?

CHAPTER TWENTY FOUR
Voodoo and the Magic Bullet

"His life, his challenges, aren't like everybody else's his age. His life may appear easier in some ways, but when you don't know what's going on around you, you can get very lonely."

In the early years of Kyler's development we considered and participated in many different kinds of therapy treatments. I considered many of those methods to be "**voodoo**" because they made no medical sense to me. It took me some time to come to the understanding that my son's problems were not going to be solved by a pill, surgery, or any other medical procedure. Of course that was hard to swallow because with modern medicine, I would have thought doctors were on top of this stuff.

Because not all autistic kids are the same, what works for one may not work for another. So that leaves parents with all kinds of options. Some are crazier then others, but most are still out there on the fringe of "**You have gotta be kidding!**" Right across to straight out quackery. We tried everything we could financially handle. No one thing helped to the point of "curing" my sons, but we did see small amounts of improvement here and there.

There is no cure for autism. No matter what you have read or been told. It is a lifetime neurological and behavioral disability. However, there are things that have been found to help with the characteristics so that the child/person can perhaps function better.

I'll review a few of the things we tried, and say to you—try what you can afford and what is available for free from government agencies. Also, there may be autistic groups in your state that are doing things which will be beneficial to your child. Get used to putting miles behind the wheel, because some therapies will be required daily and sometimes multiple times a day. I won't share my thoughts about each one other than to say, I am always thinking, "**COO KOO.**"

Applied Behavioral Analysis (ABA): This uses behavior therapy to teach skills that kids with autism lack. It is provided in the home 30-40 hours a week and is considered the most intensive program for autism treatment.

Sound/music auditory integration: You go twice a day to a specialist who has your kid sit listening with earphones to sounds and music. This was done for two weeks twice a day.

Yoga/speech therapy: Once a week the boys go to this special yoga class and learn how to monitor and express themselves and try to relax through emotional stress.

Play therapy: Autistic kids don't know how to creatively play with toys using their imagination. So adults teach them how to do this. This can be done under the umbrella of ABA or as prescribed by other professionals. It is dedicated time on a certain task of learning.

Cranial Sacral therapy: A person slowly manipulates the bones in the child's head for an hour, helping to align his center. This slow manipulation can also be done on varying parts of the body so that the flow of energy is not blocked throughout the system.

Doctor of Osteopathic Medicine (D.O.): We met with one who was highly recommended and would start each body manipulation therapy with a prayer to God for assistance. I am a Christian and strongly believe in the power of prayer, but this D.O. took prayer to a new level. He would then massage, pull, push, bend, and stretch Kyler to stimulate the body. It was a combination of cranial sacral therapy and body manipulation.

Compression therapy: I had to learn this one so that I could do it. It takes compressing every bone/joint in the body starting with the smallest joints and moving to the whole body. I continue to do this even today with my teenage boy.

Sensory Integration: Rubbing the body of the child with a surgical washing brush. Starting with the fingers and moving up the arms to the neck, head, then down to the body. This is a means of awakening the sensory system. It also helps with focus and calming the child. This can also involve movement from various equipment, swings, balls, and exercises done with occupational therapists as well as parental supervision.

Weighted Vest or Blanket: At the suggestion of the occupational therapist we acquired a weight vest. This is a vest that has pockets all over it. You fill these pockets with small sand bags. This helps to slow the sensory system down to help with overload and to help the child focus.

Horse therapy: Weekly or more often, trips to the stables to let the child socialize with and ride horses. It is said that the horse is very in tune with special needs kids and they make a connection. It also helps to teach socialization skills to autistic children; however, this is very expensive and might not be realistic for many.

The frog swing: A form of sensory integration. We had to clear out the garage so there would be room for this contraption. It was a hook in the ceiling attached to some strong industrial bungee cords. These were then attached to a soft kind of saddle. When we first got it, Kyler would spend many hours a day jumping around the garage on it. He knew exactly where he was in space at all times so that he never hit any of the walls. It was truly amazing to watch. It calmed the sensory system.

Carabiner for spinning on a platform swing: Used for sensory integration training. A contraption I had to build into our back porch. With a strong support cross beam, I put an eye hook into the ceiling. This was attached to a carabiner that could spin freely. It was then attached to four ropes that were put into a square frame several inches off the ground. This frame was then covered with carpet so you could sit or kneel on it while holding the ropes. Kyler could spin as fast as we could spin him until we got tired. He would **never** get dizzy. After getting off it he would walk like normal. Literally 30 seconds for me and I was falling down dizzy and sick to my stomach. Truly, seeing is believing. This is for the sensory system.

Zrii health drink: I was told this stuff would cure my son. This was a multi-level marketing product that was the "miracle juice." I persuaded a distributer to give me a one-month supply of the product and I would use it religiously with my son. I told him if it worked, I would work with him to sell this stuff and Kyler would be a poster child. After a week on the product my son got so out of control we had to stop it cold. It took several weeks for him to get his system back to his normal. I'm not saying this stuff does not work; it just did not work for our son.

Juice Plus: Cleans out the digestive system so that the chemicals will be balanced in the body.

Pure oxygen therapy: Having your child sit for an hour at a time in a hermetically sealed tank, and then having a doctor pump in pure oxygen.

Social Skills Groups: Autistic children do not pick up on social cues just by observation. They must be taught every nuance. These are groups with and without special needs kids. The instructor teaches step by step, what to say, how to say it, what facial expressions mean, and personal space issues. Basically everything that most of us just pick up through our peer groups on what is right and wrong and what is acceptable or not.

The list goes on and on. I will list below a few that I have not covered above and have no real experience with. Remember, many of these have no scientific proof that they work, but you will meet many therapists that will swear by them. Many people will try them with varied amounts of success and/or no success at all. I have come to learn these things are like fixing a car. You start with the least expensive part when trying to find something you're not sure about, then move up the financial ladder of expense until you find the problem. My wife and I refer to this as "the checklist." We have worked through it over the years. Some of it has worked; some hasn't, and some we just don't know, but we never stop trying. You can do your own research on all of the therapies listed above and below. There is lots of information on the Internet both pro and con, but it's up to you to make your own choices. Remember you can find research to support any method. That is why it is up to you to do your homework and choose what is right for your family.

Pivotal response therapy
Aversion therapy
Communication interventions
Son-Rise therapy
TEACCH
Qigong Massage
Neuro feedback therapy
Patterning therapy
Packing therapy
Special Oils

Diets, Diets, Diets. Many different diets out there claim they will cure autism. You have to be the judge for yourself.

Let me once again stress that many of these therapies are not clinically tested and proven methods of treatment for autism. But we have and do engage in some of them even now as our sons are teenagers and growing into adults.

Here is a list of websites that you might find helpful. Again, every person with autism is different, so you may be looking for different support or information. It is good to look at several different opinions.

> autismcenter.org:
>> *This site is for the Southern Arizona Research and Resource Center. (I would devour their quarterly magazine. It was filled with useful information.)*
>
> Autismspeaks.org
> Myautism.com
> Autism.org
> Autismkey.com
> Autismsciencefoundation.org
> Nationalautismassociation.org
> Myautismteam.com

CHAPTER TWENTY FIVE
COMPREHENSION & CONFUSION

"He wants to please you but he has to understand what he needs to do to please you, and if you're not clear or change the presentation of your message, he will fail and you will be frustrated."

After all the Voodoo and therapy that is out there and all the different things we have tried, I still have to accept the fact that my sons are autistic. They will never be like other kids no matter how hard I try to make them, how much therapy I can get for them, nor how many voodoo sessions they undergo. They do not comprehend like you and I, nor will they ever be seen, accepted, and understood in the world like a "normal" person. That is one of the problems with autism. The children look so normal that people cannot accept that anything is wrong with them. We had a psychologist tell us that is the discrimination we face. Autistic people are discriminated against because they don't have any features that scream special needs. Because of that, people have no patience with them and just assume that their behaviors are faked and done on purpose to get out of work or to bother others.

These things being said, I do not stop trying to make them "normal." There is still a small part of me that is struggling to push them across the line to being "normal," or maybe it's me doing what I always have when it comes to my boys: push, push, and then push some more. I try to teach them and coach them and demand from them the very best they can be so that their lives can be as full as possible, whatever that is. I hate to admit it but sometimes I get VERY frustrated with them when they do not comprehend something I'm trying to teach them, and we have gone over things again and again. As you will see from a few examples I will share here, patience is a virtue I do not always master, but I do try. Heaven knows I try.

I took the boys and my 9-year-old daughter, Shea, on a fishing trip into a remote area of the mountains in Arizona. We were with a group of about 15 people who were going to be strewn across 5 to 6 miles of very rugged river conditions. I knew that Koleden would not be able to cover much land due to the very difficult terrain, but I wanted to share with them my love of nature and the outdoors. We made the arduous trek up and down a rather large mountain. The walk was only about half a mile, but the terrain was so tough that it took about 45 minutes to make it to the river and the first fishing hole. Before getting started we reviewed the safety rules about what happens if we get separated. We had been camping before, and one of my greatest fears is losing one of my kids in the wilderness. Even though I worry, I still feel I can't just shield my kids from everything. They need to be shown the world around them and be exposed to things outside of their classrooms and therapist rooms. It is my hope that these experiences will help them grow and become a few steps closer to "normal."

So here are the rules we reviewed over and over if you get lost or separated from the group: STOP, SIT DOWN, AND WAIT TO BE FOUND. Do not go looking for me, do not try to get back to camp, do not start walking up or down the river looking for someone, do not keep fishing in the river. STOP, SIT DOWN, AND WAIT TO BE FOUND. I will come and find you as soon as I notice you are missing. Most importantly: "stay next to the river." I repeated those instructions several times and in different ways. As I have said before, the boys often do not totally comprehend what I'm saying, so by restating an important message in different ways they start to get the meaning. I have learned an important step to this process. After I have given direct instructions, an additional step is needed, especially with Kyler. It is this: I ask a question or two and have him answer with a complete sentence and not a yes or no answer. That way he demonstrates to me that he understands the message. On this occasion I asked, "Kyler, how do you get back to camp if we get separated?" The reply I got floored me and I honestly got angry. His response to my question was, "Just go back up the hill to where camp is." I then asked my 9-year-old daughter the same question and she replied, "Sit down and wait for you to find me." So, frustrated and in a very sharp voice, I repeated all the previous instructions and commands with some variations to try to make sure there was 100% understanding about what to do. I then asked several more questions to ensure there was complete understanding. I worry about the boys' safety, but I look for ways to teach them about unsafe situations that may come up in their lives and how to deal with them. I don't know if I'm doing the right thing but hey, there are no manuals.

On countless occasions I have tried to teach Kyler how to help me back my truck up to the trailer and hook them together. The person in the truck follows the instructions of the person giving him directions, aligning the receiver hitch to a trailer coupler. There is not a lot of room for error in this exercise, as you are trying to align a two-inch round ball on the back of the truck with the small coupler on the front of the trailer. We have gone through this exercise many, many times, and invariably Kyler will stop me before the two points are aligned.

I can actually complete this task on my own, but I want to teach him how to help, so we go through the same exercise over and over. He tells me when to stop backing up and then gives me small directions on which way I need to turn to align the truck's ball with the trailer's coupler.

Sometimes his directions are so far off that I am two feet from the desired alignment. We then go through the signals again as to what I need him to do so that we can complete the task correctly. We try again, repeating the entire process. Sometimes we are successful, and that is a time for rejoicing, but most of the time I end up doing it myself with him watching.

Once the ball and the coupler are together, we must then complete the process of properly securing the truck and trailer together. It is very important that every step is completed from a safety standpoint, so even if Kyler completes the job, I still must inspect all his work. He usually will forget one or two items every time. Here is what is entailed in the final steps of securing the trailer to the truck: lock down the trailer coupler to the ball; attach two safety chains from the trailer to the truck; plug in the trailer lights; attach the safety brake wire to the truck. That does not seem like a lot to do, but for Kyler, I might as well be teaching him how to build a spaceship. I do not know if there are just too many steps for him to remember. What I do know is that he can't see the unsecured chains one time, then another time he won't notice the lock on the ball. It always seems to be something different that he misses. So far, he has never done it correctly in all the times we have coupled the truck to the trailer. I will continue to try and never give up on my son.

So you may ask why I put myself through this over and over again? I really can't honestly answer that question. When he was younger, and I first started trying to teach him this task, it would make me absolutely crazy that he could not figure it out. I mean how hard could it be to give me directions and then lower the trailer coupler onto the ball? I would get frustrated with him when he would direct me to back the truck up only to have it bump into the trailer or have me so far off that I would have to start all over. Sometimes, when I was in a hurry, I would snap at him for not getting me even close; I regret those times. There would be other times I would look at the connections and say, "You missed something," and he would look and look at the hitch and trailer and not see the hanging chain or unsecured brake wire. I would give him a verbal cue, and then he might or might not see the step he missed.

Years have passed and we still have not mastered this maneuver, but I have developed much more patience and have to hope that one day Kyler will get it. One day all the parts of this task will click in his brain....or not. Much of life with Kyler is like this, whether it is doing the dishes, washing the car, stacking the wood, cleaning his room, or playing golf. Kyler's inability to see detail becomes clear to me when the steps needed to complete a task are often just out of reach for his understanding, comprehension, or memory.

Again, I come back to what people see when they look at Kyler—a normal looking kid that should be able to do things just like everyone else his age. What I see and experience is a young man, that try as he might, just does not see everything we see, a young man who does not understand how to follow a set of given directions very well. That is not because he does not want to or because he is being lazy, but because his brain is just wired a bit differently than ours.

CHAPTER TWENTY SIX
I'M STILL DECODING THEM

*"It pains me to hear he's bullied at school and on the bus.
How do I protect him? How do I save him? I can't be with
him every minute of the day. What do I do?"*

When Kyler was 15-years-old, the remake of "True Grit" with Jeff
Bridges was released on video. Now if you have seen this film you
know that the language, even though it is English, can be a bit hard
to understand. I was sitting with Kyler, watching this western tale,
just enjoying a movie together. About midway through the movie I
turned to Kyler and asked him if he was enjoying it. He shrugged his
shoulders and said, "Not really." I put the movie on pause and asked
him if he understood what was happening. Again he shrugged his
shoulders and shook his head. I asked him why he was still sitting
there watching a movie when he had no idea what was going on. He
said he just wanted to sit with me and be with me.

This interchange opened up a whole new thought to me. I asked
him if he understood movies better if the subtitles were on. He said
sometimes. So I pushed a bit farther and asked him what kind of
movies he did like to watch. He responded, "Megamind." I asked
him why. His response caught me off guard because his reasons for
enjoying a movie had not changed since he was a baby. He liked the
action and movement on the screen. I asked him a few questions
about the movie "Megamind" to determine what he got out of it. I was
surprised to find that he enjoyed the action but did not understand
why the main character was so unhappy with his life once he had

vanquished the hero. He did not understand the main character's desire for companionship with the investigative reporter. He could recite the general story perfectly, but the nuances of the film escaped him completely. He had seen the movie at least 50 times and only now were we having a discussion about the meaning of the movie outside of the action scenes. I asked him what he thought about while watching the movie when it was between action scenes. He thought for a second then said, "Nothing." I said, "Nothing?" He thought again for a few seconds then said, "No, just waiting for the action to start again."

So why do I tell this story? Regardless of how well it appears Kyler is progressing, it further reminds me of the limitations of his future. His inability to understand interpersonal relationships means: no wife, no children, no real friendships. These considerations are still difficult for me to accept. The things which fill my life with happiness will never be his. I worry where he will find happiness. What kinds of activities or events will bring him fullness and pleasure? Will he ever find true happiness, or will he live a life oblivious to the happiness that most people feel? As he gets older and has the ability (by virtue of his age) to make his own decisions, will he spend more time being entertained by video games, TV, or some other form of media? These thoughts haunt me daily as I pine over his future. It breaks my heart to consider his lack of fullness in life as "normal" people define it. Now I have to ask myself, "What can I do to change his fortune, improve his lot in life?" There are so many questions I must struggle with, so few answers to the unknown. Perhaps all parents have these thoughts about their offspring, but I also have two "normal" kids, so I understand those feelings as well. I assure you they are very different. Those "normal" children's personal choices will someday come into play and end up being beyond the control of the parent. That is not the case with Kyler. He is not in charge of his own destiny, primarily because this concept is beyond his comprehension.

CHAPTER TWENTY SEVEN
A GROWN MAN CRYING

"Watching young Kyler on his football team was very sad.
He would get punished for not doing things right, when in
all truth he did not understand the directions."

I was driving around town running some errands when the following event took place. It moved me so much I had to stop driving and just sit on the side of the road and listen.

I'm not often if ever moved to tears, but listening to a nationally syndicated sports talk show did just that a few years ago. Following the February 15, 2006, Jason McElwain incident, where an autistic boy scored 20 points in the closing minutes at a high school basketball game, Jim Rome did a segment where he talked about the actions of the coach and kids on the team. He also discussed how the fans at the home game reacted to the incident. It was a moving segment that introduced the rest of the show. Callers from all over the country started to call in and relate similar stories about extraordinary acts of kindness where special needs kids were made to feel normal, if only for a brief moment in their difficult lives. In almost every instance those great acts of kindness were somewhat planned. If the sporting contests were nearing the end and the outcome was clear, the special kid would get in the game. The officials had to be included in the plan because sometimes rules needed to be slightly altered. In all instances, fans made the moment very special.

Caller after caller for two hours would come on and tell stories from the point of view of the parent, official, spectator, player, or coach. As these stories would unfold I was moved to tears so badly I was unable to drive. I felt such great pain and happiness as each story was related. It made me ask myself if my sons would be treated so graciously by others in their lives. Would they instead feel nothing but pain at not being included or wanted? Would they ever participate in school sports? Would they never feel that sense of accomplishment and victory in the field of athletics? Would they ever be allowed to participate in any way on teams that required you to have a specific skill set to be included? Was that part of my life, which brought and still brings me such joy, not to be a part of my boys' lives? All those emotions came to the surface while listening to the Jim Rome show that day in my car.

This all struck closer to home in 2011. I had moved our family to the Albuquerque, New Mexico, area following a new job opportunity. This was a tough transitional time for Brenna as she was moving into her junior year. Dana and Brenna spent several days exploring the school options in the area to ensure we were doing the best we could for our kids. We settled in the community of Rio Rancho, primarily because of the positive things we had been told about the new 3 year old, V. Sue Cleveland High School. During the 2011-2012 school year, Cleveland High School posted an impressive, athletic program accumulated GPA of 3.17. Coupled with this and maybe more impressive, the school ranked 19th in the nation in overall athletics by "MAXPREPS," the pre-eminent high school sports rating system. The school won 9 New Mexico big school state championships in various sports, both for girls and boys, including the prestigious State 5-A Football Championship, ending the season a perfect 14-0.

So why does this matter? We did not choose the school for that impressive athletic record. As with all American high schools, the long held tradition of a homecoming King and Queen are chosen by the entire student body. As usual that took place in the fall of 2011, but there was something different about this class, and it was not their athletic prowess. It was their humanity and compassion. Two surprise names were nominated during the online voting. They were two barely verbal special needs kids. Both were well-liked because of their ready smiles, boundless energy, and engaging personalities. To the surprise of everyone in the school, those two special needs people were chosen by the student body to represent their school as the Homecoming King and Queen. The roar of applause at the student assembly was deafening as the administrator announced the winners of what is often just a popularity contest. Five standing ovations later, there were few dry eyes in the auditorium. Even the heralded non-emotional football coach had tears streaming down his face. That selection came as a surprise because there had not been a campaign of any sort to get those two young people selected. Voting was done online in the privacy of each student's home.

That outcome was a testament of the compassion of the entire student body for those two young people who were not beautiful in the general sense of the word but are beautiful souls and loving human beings. My daughter cried at the outpouring of support for those two special kids. It made her proud of her new school. Even the nominees who were not selected were pleased with the outcome of this unique selection. "C" and "D" represented their school well at the ceremonies. I do not know their parents, but I can imagine their heartfelt pride and appreciation for the overwhelming kindness shown to their precious children. During the homecoming football game half-time coronation, there were two more standing ovations. Many tears were seen in the crowd, tears of joy, tears of happiness, tears of pride.

Being the father of autistic or special needs children brings all those kinds of stories into a unique focus and perspective. Only those of us with such children can understand and feel deep in our hearts, minds, and souls the true blessings that experiences like those provide for our children.

Many years ago I asked my wife this question: Are we doing the right thing trying to take Kyler and Koleden out of their world of oblivion? Prior to the age of 10, they did not recognize when someone was mean or did not like them. They had no understanding of mean kids and things said or actions done to them that were meant to hurt. I asked the question again as the boys entered junior high and high school. Have we done the right thing helping them develop to their present levels? The outward appearance of my boys would never lead anyone to think they are mentally disabled, but they are and in some ways severely so.

When I changed jobs and moved my family to a new city in a new state, the boys were going into junior high and high school respectively. I knew this would be difficult for them but how difficult I will never know. I was not there to see the effects of how they were treated at school. I sat down with the boys one day, inquiring about how their lives were going at their new schools. The ensuing answers caused me such pain and worry that I was up most of the next few nights pondering what I could do to help them cope with their difficulties. The answers never came, just more worrying and concern for their happiness. I feel some concerns and worries for my daughters, but in the end they have friends; they have positive experiences most days at school; They develop friends at church. This is not the case for my boys.

During a recent in-depth conversation with Koleden, I asked him about lunch recess period. His answer pained me because of the polar opposite of how my youth played out on the recess playground. He shared with me how he tried to play basketball and football with the other kids, but due to his lack of athletic ability and barely rudimentary understanding of both the nuances and rules of the game, the other kids would not let him play. On the rare occasion he was allowed to participate he was not given the ball. He was just on the playing field taking up space. So I asked him what he does at recess. He said, "I just walk around watching everybody. Sometimes I talk to the teachers." I asked him if he had any friends at school to play with. He considered the question then responded, "No."

Koleden's inability to empathize and consider other's point of view will often get in the way of his having friends. At home we often refer to Koleden as the "Rules Policeman." Sports or games like football or basketball have many clear and concise rules. In the case of young athletes the games are played with rules often being used only as guidelines and only the most flagrant flaunting or obvious breaking of the rules are applied. These are the gray areas that, though the rule is clearly stated, the official's call could go either way. For example—in football, I would venture to say the offensive line holds someone somewhere on every pass play. But do we see a flag on every play? No! The officials make judgement calls on each play based on how serious the offense was and if it directly impacts the play.

Those concepts are impossible for my boys to comprehend. Living in a black or white world when it comes to decision makes living in their world difficult. So on the playground when someone breaks a rule or pushes a rule to the gray area, Koleden gets upset. He invariably goes to the teacher for rectification, thus alienating him from his peers because he is a tattle tale. This is repeated daily and most days he is left with two results. First and most importantly he becomes an outcast from the other students. Second, the teachers tire of this cycle, and who could blame them? It is the child crying "wolf."

Koleden's obsession, and I do mean obsession, with rules and his interpretation of them is unbendable. For years we have counseled him in various ways. "Let things go." "Enjoy playing the game." "It will make you friends." "You don't always have to be right." "People will like you better if you don't tattle all the time." Our suggestions were to no avail. He is like an addict, a compulsive person, a stutterer, he cannot control himself. He must enforce the rule, and if he cannot enforce the rule with his peers, he must tattle. Most of the time his action, his complaint, his lack of control, will not benefit him, but 100 out of 100 times he will pursue that course of action. In the end it does not and has never ended well for my boy, but he continues on the same path, and I worry for him every day as he leaves for school. Will this be the day he comes home beaten and bloodied because he is so different? There is no question he is bullied and belittled most days, even if only in small ways. It happens and there is very little we can do to curtail it. The school definitely does not.

Koleden did not have the advantage of the thousands of hours of therapy that Kyler had. That was definitely a disadvantage for him and will ultimately be a huge negative factor in his life. He was not able to get early intervention because he was late-onset-autism, and we just did not have the money to pay for all the therapy he needed. He was not trained how to socialize and how to deal with emotion as was his brother. He was not taught how to recognize facial expressions and deal with frustrations. In a nutshell all the advantages that Kyler had in regard to therapies and habilitation skills were never provided for Koleden beyond what we could do as parents. Suffice it to say, we will always be haunted by the fact that we could not do as much for this son. As everything went right and fell into place for Kyler, it was just the opposite for Koleden.

I understand in my head why he has NO friends, but my heart hurts for him. My soul suffers to know that my boy is an outcast, a pariah. As I have mentioned, I have coached him in Little League baseball. One reason for this is so I can control his compulsiveness and his need to be right, to be the "Rules Policeman." I try to monitor his every move, his every interaction with his teammates, his every retort or response to a situation. I can often cut him off from inappropriate responses, flashes of anger, or his need to tattle. I can just say his name in a certain tone and often get him to stop in his tracks, but over the course of a practice he gets so much built up behind his dam of emotion that he needs to burst and let some out. Then he blurts out something that makes his peers stop and notice and probably think he is weird or off his rocker.

He does not cuss or swear; we do not allow that, but he will have to correct the actions of another person in an aggressive way, or to tattle to another coach or adult, looking for redress which never comes. He must tell and therein lies his greatest social mountain to climb. Will we ever get there? I don't know, but will I ever stop trying? No, I can't, because he's my boy and I love him. I wish I could protect him by going everywhere with him, monitoring his every move and action, and helping him make better decisions in his people skills. I know I can't, but deep in my heart while I lie awake in the darkness of night, I wish I could. I try to find solutions in my head that never come. I ache inside just trying to guess what his life is like walking around the perimeter of the playground, on the edge of existence, looking inward to the playground, hearing the laughing playing kids, and being unable to understand. "Why can't I be part of that? Why can't I have friends? Why don't people like me? Why do I have to be autistic?"

What will his life be like? Will he find a girl that makes him happy? Will he have friends he can confide in? Will he be able to get a job? Will he...Will he?...Will he......? And I again fall asleep with no answers, no plan, just a knowledge that I will always love, teach, and advocate for him to the best of my abilities.

For the many times I see and hear "Defeat," I lie there silently, under the cover of darkness, with tears running down my cheeks wondering if I can get up again and face the challenges of being the father my sons need. I continue to fall and make mistakes and I continue to force myself to find the will to get up and try again. To realize that "winning is no more than ....to rise each time [I] fall," to admit to myself that win or lose I will not quit. This race in life, my journey with Kyler and Koleden, is worth the pain of falling down and finding the strength within me to get up and finish the race. I have learned to embrace the unique journey I am on. I love my sons and am grateful they are MY BOYS.

APPENDIX I

KYLER'S OPINION ON BEING AUTISTIC:
TYPED BY DANA FROM A RECORDING BY KYLER (AGE 11)

I don't really like being autistic, because I don't like taking pills. I don't like having to go and take my medicine at night when I am playing and having fun. I don't like taking medicine in the morning. I have never been made fun of because I am autistic, but I know that I will be someday. There will be some older kids that will make fun of me. I am always hoping that someone will be there for me and protect me. I probably act funny or sometimes I lose control of my temper and actions. My body just sometimes has a mind of its own.

I would explain autism as, " I have to take pills to control my hyperness and myself. It is hard to learn things because I am so hyper. Sometimes I go into my own world and I miss a lot that is said or explained. I have a really hard time understanding what people are saying, because sometimes I just don't hear them. I am in my own place. School is sometimes very hard for me becasue I go into my own world."

APPENDIX II

*"In his entire life he has had only a few friends and
ultimately they always have outgrown him
which leaves him very sad"*

Why my dad is the best ever.

I really love my dad because he has helped me in so many ways that
no one could imagine. Everytime I see him leave, I miss him. He
has allways helped me understand things that include using tools to
build. I don't know what I would do without him. I have known him
as my best friend and also my teacher. I can't wait until we move, so
I can be with him everyday, so then I will see him after work and
make his life more fun when he comes home. It has been so hard
without him because I am a jerk when he's not around. I need to be
better with my siblings. I wish I knew how Koleden almost always
annoys me, and I feel like he gets away with it. Mom always says
he does not get away with it. I also feel like Koleden likes to pick
on me and that's why I pick on him back. I love yu so much dad, in
ways that you could not think of. You are the best dad I've ever had
in my entire life.

LOVE, KYLER

Note: I was living in Santa Fe and my family was in Tucson when Kyler wrote this. Prior to this 8-months, I had been commuting from St. Louis to Tucson for 9-months. So I had only been seeing my family one weekend every 3 weeks. It was a hard time for all of us.

APPENDIX III

KYLER'S OPINION ON BEING AUTISTIC: WRITTEN BY KYLER (AGE 15)

"He looks normal. He's 15 years old, 5'10",145 lbs. The problem is he has the mind of a nine or ten-year-old from a maturity standpoint."

I'm a 15 year old autistic boy. Being autistic to me is a hard life because it is harder to learn than everybody else, and also everybody thinks it's easier because it's easy work for them, but to me it's a little bit of both. I don't like to take meds every single day because it makes me feel like I'm not like everyone else. But I know I have to take them because I will go crazy and out of control. Going out of control means I'm hyper active and have energy people would not normally have in them.

Another reason I don't like being autistic is because most of the time I don't understand what people are saying or what they are talking about. Another thing is learning is harder than it is for everyone else. It is hard because I try to learn and I end up not being able to understand. Then I get frustrated and start having a meltdown. I'm a really good reader and speller but I don't understand what I am reading. Sometimes when I talk with my brother he gets very frustrated with me, because I don't understand what he is trying to tell me, or I don't understand the subject. People at school think it is easy for me to learn because it was easy work for them, but not for me. Just because I can write or talk doesn't mean I understand what people are saying. One thing that really scares me is when people are yelling at me. I'm not afraid that I'm going to get hit, but it scares me in a way I can't describe. I like having a friend that I can trust, like Nathan, because he knows that I can't understand. He knows that I need to take meds. He knows that I can get outta control, and Nathan accepts me for who I am. I like playing sports because I get to use my energy so I can be controllable. I kinda know the rules and I kinda don't know the rules. It takes me some time to learn the rules to any game.

For me I think being autistic can be hard if you let it. It can be easy if you don't let it become hard. I've been hit 3 times in the same eye. I also got a brain bleed from getting hit in the head with a baseball from the fastest pitcher in the league. I have so much trouble. With my siblings I wish I could be better. I now have my dad to call on the phone.

If I ever need him it is so great that I can always contact my dad. If I need or want to talk to him I love calling my dad so I can make his life a little bit better. I don't always enjoy being autistic, but I just need to go with it sometimes, which is a very good attitude to have. There are times when I hate being autistic and there are also times when I get dangerously angry and I can end up hurting other people and myself. It scares me.

—Kyler (age 15)

APPENDIX IV

KOLEDEN'S OPINION ON BEING AUTISTIC:
WRITTEN BY KOLEDEN (AGE 13)

"He wants to be included with normal kids; he just doesn't understand what the social cues are."

Hi, I'm Koleden Bayardo. My feeling on being autistic is that it sucks because I have a hard time learning. Well, being autistic is not easy. I get bullied a lot. I have trouble paying attention in class and I have troble making friends. Well, people think it's not fair because I have easier textbooks and lessons. But to me they're kinda both. My problem with being autistic is that I look normal but I'm autistic. I act weird and I do weird things. You might think being autistic is easy but it isn't. It's actually quite hard to me. The problem with my old P.E. coach-- he made me run. But the thing is I didn't remember to put on the health sheet that I have a deformed foot. It's like having 2 left feet and 2 right feet anyway I'm lucky I didn't get injured from running too much. It hurts when I run or walk too much. I have to swim to get exercise cause it doesn't put pressure on my foot or hip so it doesn't hurt.

Being autistic means like I have trouble doing stuff that other people can do easily. But it doesnt mean I cant do things that other people cant do. Other people can have focus in class and they dont have energy like I do. But I do have trouble doing homework and other things. I kinda feel glad and sad about being autistic sometimes. I feel glad because it helps me to get stuff done. I get more help. I need that to do my work. I feel sad because some people think I am ordinary and I dont understand the things they understand. I look like them but I am not like them. Kids make fun of me at lunch. I do not like it. It makes me sad when I want to play basketball with them but they won't let me because they say I'm weird. I cry. I don't understand what I do that is different. it seems people want to hurt me or make me mad or sad. I dont understand. Rules are important to me. Teachers dont help me and that makes me very angry.

My weaknesses are paying attention, being calm, my temper, doing work, I chew on my fingers when I am stressed or nervous or bored. I like the smell of them. It calms me down but kids think that is weird.

My strengths are video games, building with legos part by part with and without instructions, and being quiet in class.

I don't like swimming on a swim team, loud noises, spiders, lots of people, people who are rude, or people who cuss.

I like video games, legos, camping, fishing, swimming for fun, watching tv, walking in circles, smelling my fingers.

I want to be a computer engineer because it gives a good pay and I like building things.

—Koleden (age 13)

APPENDIX V

An Oldest Sibling's View of Her Autistic Brothers: Written by Brenna (Age 17)

There are many pros and cons to having brothers with special needs. Just like anything that is hard and long going, there are times when I want to give up because it gets too hard to bear. There are times where I think, "Woe is me and why me?" But as both my parents have pointed out to me during those times, I'm throwing myself a pity party that does not help anyone or accomplish anything but make me feel bad. I'm a teenager.

I have known no other way of life. I don't know what a "normal" family is. I have had to take on more responsibility than most kids my age. Not only because my dad was the oldest of 8 in a Hispanic family, but because my brothers needed me. And there are times when I envy those families who don't have to worry about medications, therapists, doctors, shrinks, temper tantrums, etc. There are times when I wish I had not been given the responsibilities I have. But I wouldn't trade my life for anything. Because Kyler was diagnosed when I was four years old, I have had parenting skills drilled into my head. Whenever he would start screaming I was taught to completely ignore his tantrums, not to acknowledge him until he said please or stopped screaming. I was taught to be the adult.

I went to the therapists where I saw my brother "playing." He had those big people that were at the time teaching him how to play, but I was four, five, and six years old. How was I supposed to know that my little brother didn't know how to play? How was I supposed to know that he was being taught how to play? For all I knew, those adults wanted to play with him and not me.

As my dad has said, I managed to get forgotten for a time. I was subconsciously aware of the fact that I was getting set aside, that Kyler was getting more attention than I was. I couldn't take it out on Kyler; I loved him too much. So I took it out on dogs and my eating habits. One morning I woke up terrified of dogs, so terrified it was labeled a phobia of dogs. It could have been the size of a puppy and I would run and scream to someone or go someplace where I could get away from it. As for my eating habits, I would only eat what Kyler would eat.

I had to grow up the moment my parents found out that Kyler was autistic. I had to ignore Kyler's constant screaming, go help get him when he ran off, and protect him from the mean people of the world. I learned early that people are mean and ruthless and cruel at times. I got into fights for him. I would come home with black eyes for him. I was his safety blanket, the one he went crying to when people were mean to him. I am his protector.

When Koleden was diagnosed, I can remember how devastated my mom was. But both of us had to step up to the challenge. I was 10 at that time. I didn't quite realize how much having not 1 but 2 brothers with autism would impact my life. For me, it was just something else I had to live with. I didn't have as good a comprehension of what it would mean for the future because I already had one autistic brother.... what was so wrong with having two? It can't be much harder, right? Wrong. Because Dad was a workaholic, it was Mom that had to be the rock, and I subconsciously filled in the spot of being her support.

My brothers and sister mean so much to me. I was/am the protector, the 3rd parent, second mom, and there are times when I want to turn it off. There are times when I want to give up and say "screw it," the kids don't care. I am doing so much for them that they can't see anything I am doing. It is ALWAYS my fault. I will be driving to seminary (a church early morning class) or school with Kyler, and he will say something that just ticks me off. I want to be mean sometimes. I want to make them feel bad, as wrong as that sounds, and sometimes I do. But I can never bring myself to go beyond scolding them. I can never bring myself to be mean to them because I just can't. It isn't in me to be mean to them. Well, maybe to my sister.

I know that people think I am bossy and rude towards my brothers. But they know nothing. They don't understand the things I go through everyday. Temper tantrums, fighting, medicine, no comprehension of anything anyone is saying, only certain foods, no social skills, anger, favoritism, and judgement from others either towards me or my brothers. They judge me before they know that I am being the opposite of mean and rude to my brothers. I am loving and caring for them more than these people could comprehend. I am trying to teach and help my brothers get through social situations that they can't understand. I am parenting them—A habit I have tried to break, but as my mom pointed out to me, it is not a breakable habit this late in my life. I'm only 17, I know, but parenting skills have been turned on since Kyler was three. It has been drilled into my head for 14 years and is not something that I can turn off. People can't even begin to understand how I have to treat my siblings, carefully, patiently, patiently, and even more patiently.

There are times when I feel I am a horrible sister. I lose my temper. I scold them when they don't even understand what I am scolding them for. I get mad or hurt when they say something they didn't know was inappropriate at the time. I feel like if I were not a parent personality I could be a better sister, and I could have a different relationship with my siblings...but if that were the case, would it be a good change? I will never know. I may have been a worse sibling if that would have been the case.

Having special needs siblings tests your patience, your sanity, and in my case caused me to grow up and mature and be the protector. It has caused some psychological damage I think. Because I am the oldest I already have certain qualities and responsibilities, but because of the situation, they were magnified in both positive and negative ways. My brothers are brutally honest. There is no going around the bush, whatever they say they mean. This can be a really hurtful thing...but also something to learn from when they tell you how they feel. And in my opinion, the hardest thing of being a sibling to a special needs kid is that they don't get parented the same way. The excuse "They're autistic" is something heard quite often. They do not get punished like I would, and they don't have to do certain things like I did when I was their age. They aren't expected to do as much as me because "they're autistic." It doesn't seem fair at times, but then I guess it isn't fair for them either. It all depends on the perspective and state of mind you are in at the time to think whether it's fair or not.

You need to have somewhere or something that makes you happy. Something that makes you forget about the worries of the day, the home troubles. Something that is yours and yours alone. Swimming is my haven. It is where I let go of what happens during the day and forget all my worries. It is where I can be Brenna, and not Kyler's older sister.

Now believe it or not, there are some pros to having special needs brothers. As much as growing up with them stinks, it is beneficial. You mature faster, which will help you get through your teenage life easier. They love you unconditionally. They will always love you.

They may not show it or say that they love you, but in their actions and the little things they do, I assure you there is love somewhere in there. Koleden, who shows no emotions at all, came into my room the other night to give me a goodnight hug. Usually these are quick, but that one was long and came with 5 kisses to my face. I was stunned but then so touched because....I know he loves me. What 13 year old brother would give his 17 year old sister kisses before going to bed....Like he would his mom.

My brothers are pretty obedient, which comes in handy sometimes. I learned and have more patience in my life than I think a lot of other teenagers my age have. I have seen a side to life that not many other people get to see, and I hope they never have to. Whenever I am upset, Kyler and Koleden will try and comfort me. Whether it's giving me a hug or holding me while I cry. They tell me I am beautiful on Sunday when I'm getting ready for church. They tell me I'm gorgeous when I'm in my pajamas. They give me hugs and kisses before bed. They welcome me when I come home. They accidentally call me mom on occasion. They are hilarious in their own way. They come to me whenever they are scared at night. They ask me why mommy is sad when they are too scared to ask her. They tell me when they are scared of Dad and ask me to help them feel better. When I'm sick, Koleden will go out of his way to make sure I'm comfortable and feel better. Whenever I go away for any period of time, I come home to attack hugs from all of my siblings yelling, "Brennie, Brennie, Brennie!" Those are things that "normal" brothers probably would never do once they reach 11.

Because of Kyler's diagnosis, I was able to live in one city for 16 years of my life. Had Kyler not been diagnosed, we would have moved many times in the past 14 years. My dad became a better person because of my brother's diagnosis. Like Mom and I, he had to step up to the plate in certain ways. He has grown a lot because of the boys. He may have screwed up with me at times but I like to think that I turned out pretty darn all right.

I have gotten the opportunity to be around so many different specialists in many fields that work with special needs kids that I am very familiar with different diagnosis. I am planning on further investigating the subject so that I may choose a Major having to do with special-ed kids when I attend college. Because I have two autistic brothers, I am able to be patient and have a gravitational pull to and from other special needs kids that aren't my brothers. I also have more hand's-on experience than most people going into the field.

I leave for college soon. The kids have said multiple times how they don't want me to go off and leave. It breaks my heart because I am torn between staying home or going away. I love my siblings dearly and will miss them terribly but I need to get away from the house, start my own life.

Having two autistic brothers takes its toll because you're the SIBLING. You are not the parent as much as we sometimes feel. You feel it's your responsibility to take care of them and help them and try not to let them embarrass themselves. But you need to "give them some rope."

Living with them isn't an impossibility, and it's not a curse. It's a blessing in disguise, because once you're gone, you will have certain lessons, traits and experiences to lean on when you become a parent of your own.

—Brenna (age 17)

APPENDIX VI

A Youngest Sibling's View of Her Autistic Brothers: Written by Shea (Age 11)

Well, having two autistic brothers is really hard. They are hard because they don't really understand me, like if they want to leave me alone, it's just really hard to get them away. But I have to deal with it because they are my brothers and I love them.

It's hard to have brothers that are angry a lot. I mean I push buttons which is kinda a habit for me and sometimes I don't mean to but other times I do. Kyler—well, he doesn't understand to leave me alone or not to. I always try to make them laugh, but it's very hard to make Koleden laugh. It's very easy to make Kyler laugh because I just have to make funny faces.

Koleden is always hard to have a conversation with, a good one, and it's always hard to play a game with him because I mean I try but it always goes wrong. Sometimes we try to get along and he always wants to play guns and stuff and I always have to be a boy and it's very hard to. When you're in a bad conversation (argument) he never stops talking. He is always a motor mouth and it's very hard to calm him down. Sometimes me and Kyler gang up on him and it's very mean and I don't realize it at the time. I try to calm him down a lot afterwards but it doesn't go over well. Whenever I try to speak to calm him down he always tries to keep on talking (yelling), and I get frustrated and just yell "Koleden!" but he just keeps going and talking.

He has tics that I dislike, like sniffing his fingers and sniffing in general. He smacks his lips together when he eats which is very hard for me because I just don't like it. Kyler does it too. Because I have a lot of pet peeves around them, the boys get angry at me for being upset about their tics that they can't control. I can't control my not liking their tics so we are constantly fighting over that. I have learned to eat at different times than them.

Koleden gets angry very easily. Most of the time I try to leave him alone because I don't want to get in a mad conversation (argument) with him. Sometimes when he is mad at Kyler I try to calm him down. It's just he never stops talking. He just keeps going and going and going and he complains that I just keep saying please stop and I say please. He likes to get me in trouble a lot. When he is doing something wrong I go to mom and he doesn't stay in one place. He always comes with me to defend himself so that he can say he wasn't doing anything wrong, and he then stays. I try to lock him out before he can get in the room. Mom says not to lock it.

Koleden annoys me a lot and I try to deal with it. I don't know why I was chosen to be here. I don't know why I was chosen to be their sister because I have a hard time with them but I try. I have to protect him from people and Koleden always thinks I am going to embarrass him. I mean I try but it's too hard to protect him when he doesn't want me to because I'm his little sister. It's very hard.

I don't know why people are so mean, but they make it very hard. I don't know what it's like to be autistic, all I know is what it's like to be normal. Well I do have ADHD [Attention Deficit Disorder.]

A lot of people don't understand Koleden. I don't even understand him most of the time. There are so many people that don't know what happens and how he understands things. I don't know when he is in trouble because he never tells me, he never comes to me. He is not like Kyler is to Brenna. I can't be there all the time to help him in school. He got bullied last year. I wish I was there to help him, but I wasn't. I was in 5th grade and he was in 6th which meant we were in different schools. Those kids that bullied him don't know what happened or understand him at all. They just think he is a nerd and they don't like him which is sad because a lot of people don't understand special needs kids but they all need help. They all need friends. Think if it was you. You would have a hard time being without friends. All I am saying is give it a try. I mean sure it would be hard being friends with them being autistic but at least you tried and at least you didn't give up. They all need friends, I mean they don't need everybody in school. My sister, she had Kyler, she still has him, but she always protected him, she always was there, he always came to her. A lot of people made fun of her, but she didn't care, she was protecting Kyler. She was protecting family.

If you have a special needs person in your family, you should help them out as well. Even if people make fun of you because you have to protect your family. I love my family even though they are hard to live with sometimes and make me mad. They also can make me laugh.

—Shea (age 11)

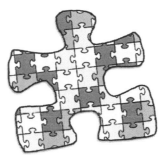

Autism: A Dad's Journey

www.autismadadsjourney.com

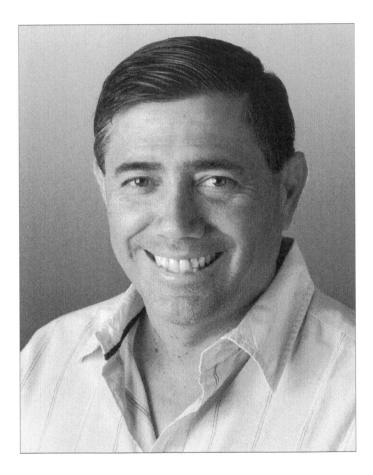

About the Author

Luis Bayardo is a father of four: two girls, and two boys who are both autistic. Devoted to his family, he has been married to Dana Nymeyer for 25 years. The oldest of eight children, he grew up in rural Arizona and left home right after high school to serve a two-year mission in South Africa for his church. Upon completing his mission Luis lived in California, Kansas, England, and the Isle of Man, and went on to receive a degree in Hospitality Management.

Luis has been in the service industry since the late 1980's and currently works as a General Manager in Santa Fe, New Mexico in the Hotel Industry. He is also an active member in his community and in his church. Convivial and easy going, Luis makes friends wherever he goes, and enjoys coaching sports, reading books, traveling, and spending time with his family. Currently, Luis finds additional fulfillment in his position as a baseball umpire where he works junior high up through Minor League professional baseball.